Diagnosis and Management of Chronic Liver Diseases

Editor

ANNE M. LARSON

MEDICAL CLINICS OF NORTH AMERICA

www.medical.theclinics.com

Consulting Editors
DOUGLAS S. PAAUW
EDWARD R. BOLLARD

January 2014 • Volume 98 • Number 1

ELSEVIER

1600 John F. Kennedy Boulevard • Suite 1800 • Philadelphia, Pennsylvania, 19103-2899

http://www.theclinics.com

MEDICAL CLINICS OF NORTH AMERICA Volume 98, Number 1
January 2014 ISSN 0025-7125, ISBN-13: 978-0-323-28712-8

Editor: Jessica McCool
Developmental Editor: Yonah Korngold

© **2014 Elsevier Inc. All rights reserved.**

This periodical and the individual contributions contained in it are protected under copyright by Elsevier, and the following terms and conditions apply to their use:

Photocopying
Single photocopies of single articles may be made for personal use as allowed by national copyright laws. Permission of the Publisher and payment of a fee is required for all other photocopying, including multiple or systematic copying, copying for advertising or promotional purposes, resale, and all forms of document delivery. Special rates are available for educational institutions that wish to make photocopies for non-profit educational classroom use. For information on how to seek permission visit www.elsevier.com/permissions or call: (+44) 1865 843830 (UK)/(+1) 215 239 3804 (USA).

Derivative Works
Subscribers may reproduce tables of contents or prepare lists of articles including abstracts for internal circulation within their institutions. Permission of the Publisher is required for resale or distribution outside the institution. Permission of the Publisher is required for all other derivative works, including compilations and translations (please consult www.elsevier.com/permissions).

Electronic Storage or Usage
Permission of the Publisher is required to store or use electronically any material contained in this periodical, including any article or part of an article (please consult www.elsevier.com/permissions). Except as outlined above, no part of this publication may be reproduced, stored in a retrieval system or transmitted in any form or by any means, electronic, mechanical, photocopying, recording or otherwise, without prior written permission of the Publisher.

Notice
No responsibility is assumed by the Publisher for any injury and/or damage to persons or property as a matter of products liability, negligence or otherwise, or from any use or operation of any methods, products, instructions or ideas contained in the material herein. Because of rapid advances in the medical sciences, in particular, independent verification of diagnoses and drug dosages should be made.

Although all advertising material is expected to conform to ethical (medical) standards, inclusion in this publication does not constitute a guarantee or endorsement of the quality or value of such product or of the claims made of it by its manufacturer.

Medical Clinics of North America (ISSN 0025-7125) is published bimonthly by Elsevier Inc., 360 Park Avenue South, New York, NY 10010-1710. Months of publication are January, March, May, July, September, and November. Business and editorial offices: 1600 John F. Kennedy Boulevard, Suite 1800, Philadelphia, PA 19103-2899. Periodicals postage paid at New York, NY, and additional mailing offices. Subscription prices are USD $255.00 per year (US individuals), $471.00 per year (US institutions), $125.00 per year (US Students), $320.00 per year (Canadian individuals), $612.00 per year (Canadian institutions), $200.00 per year (Canadian and foreign students), $390.00 per year (foreign individuals), and $612.00 per year (foreign institutions). To receive student/resident rate, orders must be accompanied by name of affiliated institution, date of term, and the signature of program/residency coordinator on institution letterhead. Orders will be billed at individual rate until proof of status is received. Foreign air speed delivery is included in all Clinics' subscription prices. All prices are subject to change without notice. **POSTMASTER:** Send address changes to *Medical Clinics of North America*, Elsevier Health Sciences Division, Subscription Customer Service, 3251 Riverport Lane, Maryland Heights, MO 63043. **Customer Service: Telephone: 1-800-654-2452** (U.S. and Canada); **1-314-447-8871** (outside U.S. and Canada). **Fax:** 314-447-8029. **E-mail: journalscustomerserviceusa@elsevier.com** (for print support); **journalsonlinesupport-usa@elsevier.com** (for online support).

Reprints. For copies of 100 or more of articles in this publication, please contact the Commercial Reprints Department, Elsevier Inc., 360 Park Avenue South, New York, NY 10010-1710. Tel.: 212-633-3874; Fax: 212-633-3820; E-mail: reprints@elsevier.com.

Medical Clinics of North America is also published in Spanish by McGraw-Hill Interamericana Editores S. A., P.O. Box 5-237, 06500 Mexico, D.F., Mexico.

Medical Clinics of North America is covered in *MEDLINE/PubMed (Index Medicus), Current Contents, ASCA, Excerpta Medica, Science Citation Index,* and *ISI/BIOMED.*

Printed in the United States of America.

PROGRAM OBJECTIVE
The goal of the *Medical Clinics of North America* is to keep practicing physicians up to date with current clinical practice by providing timely articles reviewing the state of the art in patient care.

TARGET AUDIENCE
All practicing physicians and other healthcare professionals.

LEARNING OBJECTIVES
Upon completion of this activity, participants will be able to:
1. Review considerations for liver transplant during the management of chronic liver disease.
2. Recognize treatment options for nonalcoholic fatty liver disease.
3. Discuss management of end-stage liver disease.

ACCREDITATION
The Elsevier Office of Continuing Medical Education (EOCME) is accredited by the Accreditation Council for Continuing Medical Education (ACCME) to provide continuing medical education for physicians.

The EOCME designates this enduring material for a maximum of 15 *AMA PRA Category 1 Credit*(s)™. Physicians should claim only the credit commensurate with the extent of their participation in the activity.

All other health care professionals requesting continuing education credit for this enduring material will be issued a certificate of participation.

DISCLOSURE OF CONFLICTS OF INTEREST
The EOCME assesses conflict of interest with its instructors, faculty, planners, and other individuals who are in a position to control the content of CME activities. All relevant conflicts of interest that are identified are thoroughly vetted by EOCME for fair balance, scientific objectivity, and patient care recommendations. EOCME is committed to providing its learners with CME activities that promote improvements or quality in healthcare and not a specific proprietary business or a commercial interest.

The planning committee, staff, authors and editors listed below have identified no financial relationships or relationships to products or devices they or their spouse/life partner have with commercial interest related to the content of this CME activity:
Saleh Alqahtani, MD; Richele L. Corrado, MD; Rena K. Fox, MD, FACP; Andrea A. Gossard, MS, CNP; Brynne Hunter; Pushpjeet Kanwar, MD; Kris V. Kowdley, MD; Sandy Lavery; Iris W. Liou, MD; Jessica McCool; Brian J. McMahon, MD, MACP; Jill McNair; Lindsay Parnell; Santha Priya; Reena J. Salgia, MD; M.S.; Jayant A. Talwalkar, MD, MPH; Dawn M. Torres, MD; Tinsay A. Woreta, MD.

The planning committee, staff, authors and editors listed below have identified financial relationships or relationships to products or devices they or their spouse/life partner have with commercial interest related to the content of this CME activity:
Stephen A. Harrison, MD is a consultant/advisor for Nimbus Discovery and Genentech.

Anne M. Larson, MD, FACP, AGAF is on speakers bureau for Gilead, Genentech, Salix and Quintiles; has royalties/patents with UpToDate.

Amit G. Singal, MD is on Speaker's Bureau for Onyx and Bayer.

UNAPPROVED/OFF-LABEL USE DISCLOSURE
The EOCME requires CME faculty to disclose to the participants:
1. When products or procedures being discussed are off-label, unlabelled, experimental, and/or investigational (not US Food and Drug Administration (FDA) approved); and
2. Any limitations on the information presented, such as data that are preliminary or that represent ongoing research, interim analyses, and/or unsupported opinions. Faculty may discuss information about pharmaceutical agents that is outside of FDA-approved labelling. This information is intended solely for CME and is not intended to promote off-label use of these medications. If you have any questions, contact the medical affairs department of the manufacturer for the most recent prescribing information.

TO ENROLL
To enroll in the *Medical Clinics of North America* Continuing Medical Education program, call customer service at 1-800-654-2452 or sign up online at http://www.theclinics.com/home/cme. The CME program is available to subscribers for an additional annual fee of USD $267.

METHOD OF PARTICIPATION

In order to claim credit, participants must complete the following:

1. Complete enrolment as indicated above.
2. Read the activity.
3. Complete the CME Test and Evaluation. Participants must achieve a score of 70% on the test. All CME Tests and Evaluations must be completed online.

CME INQUIRIES/SPECIAL NEEDS

For all CME inquiries or special needs, please contact elsevierCME@elsevier.com.

MEDICAL CLINICS OF NORTH AMERICA

**DOWNLOAD
Free App!**

Review Articles
THE CLINICS

NOW AVAILABLE FOR YOUR iPhone and iPad

Contributors

CONSULTING EDITORS

DOUGLAS S. PAAUW, MD, MACP
Professor of Medicine, Division of General Internal Medicine, Rathmann Family Foundation Endowed Chair for Patient-Centered Clinical Education; Medicine Student Programs, Professor of Medicine, University of Washington School of Medicine, Seattle, Washington

EDWARD R. BOLLARD, MD, DDS, FACP
Professor of Medicine, Associate Dean of Graduate Medical Education, Designated Institutional Official, Department of Medicine, Penn State-Hershey Medical Center/Penn State University College of Medicine, Hershey, Pennsylvania

EDITOR

ANNE M. LARSON, MD, FACP, AGAF
Director, Swedish Liver Center, Swedish Health Services, Seattle, Washington

AUTHORS

SALEH A. ALQAHTANI, MD
Assistant Professor of Medicine, Division of Gastroenterology and Hepatology, The Johns Hopkins Hospital, Baltimore, Maryland

RICHELE L. CORRADO, MD
Department of Medicine, Walter Reed National Military Medical Center, Bethesda, Maryland

RENA K. FOX, MD, FACP
Professor of Clinical Medicine, Division of General Internal Medicine, Department of Medicine, University of California, San Francisco School of Medicine, San Francisco, California

ANDREA A. GOSSARD, MS, CNP
Cholestatic Liver Disease Study Group, Division of Gastroenterology and Hepatology, Mayo Clinic, Rochester, Minnesota

STEPHEN A. HARRISON, MD
Division of Gastroenterology, Department of Medicine, San Antonio Military Medical Center, Fort Sam Houston, Texas

PUSHPJEET KANWAR, MD
Liver Center of Excellence, Digestive Disease Institute, Virginia Mason Medical Center, Seattle, Washington

KRIS V. KOWDLEY, MD
Liver Center of Excellence, Digestive Disease Institute, Virginia Mason Medical Center, Seattle, Washington

IRIS W. LIOU, MD
Assistant Professor of Medicine, Division of Gastroenterology, Department of Medicine, University of Washington School of Medicine, Seattle, Washington

BRIAN J. MCMAHON, MD, MACP
Medical and Research Director, Liver Disease and Hepatitis Program, Alaska Native Tribal Health Consortium, Anchorage, Alaska; Research Associate, Arctic Investigations Program, Centers for Disease Control and Prevention

REENA SALGIA, MD
Senior Staff Hepatologist, Division of Gastroenterology and Hepatology, Henry Ford Hospital, Detroit, Michigan

AMIT G. SINGAL, MD, MS
Assistant Professor, Dedman Scholar of Clinical Care, Division of Digestive and Liver Diseases, University of Texas Southwestern; Harold C Simmons Cancer Center, University of Texas Southwestern Medical Center, Dallas, Texas

JAYANT A. TALWALKAR, MD, MPH
Cholestatic Liver Disease Study Group, Division of Gastroenterology and Hepatology, Mayo Clinic, Rochester, Minnesota

DAWN M. TORRES, MD
Division of Gastroenterology, Department of Medicine, Walter Reed National Military Medical Center, Bethesda, Maryland

TINSAY A. WORETA, MD
Division of Gastroenterology and Hepatology, The Johns Hopkins Hospital, Baltimore, Maryland

Contents

Serum biochemical tests play an important role in the diagnosis and management of acute and chronic liver disease. Their routine use has led to the increased detection of liver enzyme abnormalities in otherwise asymptomatic patients. These tests consist of markers of hepatocellular injury, tests of liver metabolism, and tests of liver synthetic function. Liver injury can be characterized as primarily hepatocellular versus cholestatic based on the degree of elevation of aminotransferases compared with alkaline phosphatase. A comprehensive history, physical examination, and assessment of pattern of liver injury with additional directed laboratory testing establish the cause of hepatobiliary disease in most cases.

Over 400,000 people worldwide are chronically infected with hepatitis B virus (HBV), and are at increased risk of developing hepatocellular carcinoma (HCC) and cirrhosis. HBV infected persons need regular lifelong follow-up. Candidates for antiviral therapy include patients with moderate-to-severe liver disease as determined by elevated alanine aminotransferase and/or liver biopsy and elevated HBV DNA levels above 2000 IU/mL, per evidenced-based guidelines. Pegylated interferon, tenofovir and entecavir are the first line drugs of choice for those needing treatment. All patients undergoing cancer chemotherapy or immunosuppressive therapy should be screened for hepatitis B surface antigen (HBsAg) and given HBV antiviral prophylaxis if positive.

Nonalcoholic fatty liver disease (NAFLD) remains the most common chronic liver disease in the western world and its prevalence is rising elsewhere. Among patients with NAFLD, those with nonalcoholic steato-hepatitis (NASH) represent a large potential public health concern with risk for development of cirrhosis and hepatocellular carcinoma. The ability to diagnose and treat NAFLD and NASH has improved and continues to improve as understanding of the pathogenesis of this disease develops. This article highlights the key features of NAFLD and NASH, as well as the available and future promising treatment options.

Cholestatic liver disease may involve both extrahepatic and intrahepatic bile ducts, or may be limited to one or the other. Cholestasis may be due primary bile duct disease or secondary causes such as stones or tumors. Care of the patient with cholestasis depends on identifying the probable cause, initiating appropriate treatment or intervention, and the recognition and management of potential complications.

Hereditary hemochromatosis and Wilson disease are autosomal recessive storage disorders of iron and copper overload, respectively. These metals are involved in multiple redox reactions, and their abnormal accumulation can cause significant injury in the liver and other organs. Over the last few decades clinicians have developed a much better understanding of these metals and their mechanism of action. Moreover, sophisticated molecular genetic testing techniques that make diagnostic testing less invasive are now available. This article updates and discusses the pathogenesis, diagnosis, and management of these metal storage disorders.

Patients with cirrhosis are at greatest risk for development of hepatocellular carcinoma (HCC) and should undergo semiannual surveillance using ultrasound, with or without alpha fetoprotein. Patients with positive surveillance testing should undergo contrast-enhanced MRI or 4-phase CT for diagnostic evaluation. There are therapeutic options for most patients with any tumor stage; however, treatment decisions must be individualized after accounting for degree of liver dysfunction and patient performance status. A multidisciplinary approach to care is recommended for optimal communication and treatment delivery. The aim of this review is to provide an up-to-date summary of the diagnosis and management of HCC.

Major complications of cirrhosis include the development of ascites, spontaneous bacterial peritonitis, hepatorenal syndrome, variceal hemorrhage, hepatic encephalopathy, and hepatocellular carcinoma. Careful evaluation and management of ascites and varices with judicious use of prophylactic therapy can improve survival. Diagnosis of hepatic encephalopathy can lead to appropriate intervention without protein restriction. Patients should undergo hepatocellular carcinoma surveillance routinely every 6 months. The development of any decompensating event should prompt referral to a liver transplant center.

With rising rates of end-stage liver disease and hepatocellular carcinoma, there is a growing demand for liver transplantation. The decision to allocate a liver to a patient is an extensive process in a transplant center, but the timing of initial referral for transplant evaluation will commonly be the responsibility of the primary care physician. This article discusses the indications and contraindications for liver transplantation. The criteria to determine timing of transplant referral are reviewed, and integration of these criteria into long-term management of patients with cirrhosis is emphasized.

Foreword

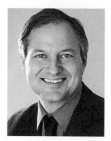

Douglas S. Paauw, MD, MACP
Consulting Editor

Liver disease is one of the most common chronic medical conditions managed by general internists. With the rise of hepatitis C over the past 40 years, the increasing frequency of NASH, and the always prevalent alcoholic liver disease, chronic liver disease has become a very common medical problem. This issue of *Medical Clinics of North America* focuses on diagnosis and management of chronic liver disease. The goal of this issue is to give current information and updates on some of the common liver problems and what the state-of-the-art workup and treatments are for these conditions. Since the development of successful liver transplantation in the 1980s, the importance of high-quality management and recognition of chronic liver disease has taken greater importance. Dr Anne Larson, one of the leading hepatologists in the United States, has put together an issue that addresses the important questions that physicians have as they manage patients with chronic liver disease.

Douglas S. Paauw, MD, MACP
University of Washington School of Medicine
Seattle, WA, USA

E-mail address:
DPaauw@medicine.washington.edu

Med Clin N Am 98 (2014) xiii
http://dx.doi.org/10.1016/j.mcna.2013.11.001
0025-7125/14/$ – see front matter © 2014 Published by Elsevier Inc.

Preface

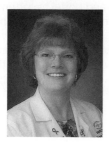

Anne M. Larson, MD, FACP, AGAF
Editor

There have been amazing advances over the last several decades in our understanding of liver disease and its treatment. In this issue of the *Medical Clinics of North America* we outline the most common diseases seen by the practicing clinician. Most liver disorders can be diagnosed by taking a meticulous history and a thorough physical examination and by recognizing the pattern of enzyme abnormalities. Second-line tests and imaging studies can then be obtained to confirm the diagnosis. This issue begins with an excellent overview by Drs Woreta and Alqahtani of the evaluation of the patient with abnormal liver tests.

Millions of persons worldwide are infected with the hepatitis C and B viruses. These patients are encountered by the clinician more frequently now than at any time in history, particularly with the influx of immigrants from countries of high endemicity. The diagnosis is crucial to optimizing patients' survival. Treatment of these viruses has continued to evolve. The field of hepatitis C virus treatment has progressed significantly over the last decade and new direct-acting antivirals are now available for treatment. These medications can provide a cure to the hepatitis C virus–infected individual. Dr McMahon offers a complete overview of the epidemiology, diagnosis, and treatment of chronic hepatitis B virus infection.

Nonalcoholic fatty liver disease (NAFLD) has become more prevalent over the last decade and mirrors the worldwide obesity epidemic. Drs Corrado, Torres, and Harrison present these alarming facts and detail the epidemiology, pathogenesis, diagnosis, and possible treatments for NAFLD. Recognizing NAFLD is essential because a portion of these patients will progress to nonalcoholic steatohepatitis with subsequent development of cirrhosis, liver cancer, end-stage liver disease, and death. As with other liver diseases, our understanding of the causes of and treatments for cholestatic and metabolic liver disease has also grown. Drs Gossard and Talwalkar discuss the diagnosis and management of the most common cholestatic liver diseases. Drs Kanwar and Kowdley present Wilson disease and hemochromatosis.

This issue of Medical Clinics of North America concludes with discussion of the complications of cirrhosis and their management. Hepatocellular carcinoma is now the sixth most prevalent cancer worldwide and the third leading cause of cancer-related death. The incidence is rising rapidly as the cirrhotic population ages. Drs Salgia

Med Clin N Am 98 (2014) xv–xvi
http://dx.doi.org/10.1016/j.mcna.2013.10.013
0025-7125/14/$ – see front matter © 2014 Elsevier Inc. All rights reserved.

and Singal provide a concise overview of the cause and management of this devastating cancer and other liver lesions. Dr Liou outlines the management of the most common complications of cirrhosis, end-stage liver disease, and portal hypertension. We end with a discussion by Dr Fox on the topic of liver transplantation and when it should be considered for these patients.

It is an extremely exciting time for those in the field of hepatology. A better understanding of these diseases and advances in treatment allow us to offer more to these patients. I would like to thank the contributors for their outstanding contributions to the field of Hepatology and this issue. I hope you enjoy reading it and find it useful in your practice.

Anne M. Larson, MD, FACP, AGAF
Swedish Liver Center
Swedish Health Services
1101 Madison Street, #200
Seattle, WA 98104-1321, USA

E-mail address:
anne.larson@swedish.org

Evaluation of Abnormal Liver Tests

Tinsay A. Woreta, MD, Saleh A. Alqahtani, MD*

KEYWORDS

- Aminotransferases • Alkaline phosphatase • Hepatocellular injury • Cholestasis
- Bilirubin metabolism

KEY POINTS

- Serum aminotransferases are sensitive markers of hepatocellular injury.
- Assessing the pattern and degree of elevation in aminotransferases can help suggest the cause of liver injury.
- Elevation in serum alkaline phosphatase occurs as a result of cholestasis, which may result from intrahepatic causes, extrahepatic obstruction, or infiltrative disorders of the liver.
- Hyperbilirubinemia may occur as the result of both hepatocellular and cholestatic injury.
- Albumin and prothrombin time are true markers of liver synthetic function.

INTRODUCTION

The use of serum biochemical tests plays an important role in the diagnosis and management of liver diseases. The routine use of such tests has led to the increased detection of liver diseases in otherwise asymptomatic patients, often providing the first clue of the presence of liver pathology. Such laboratory tests, in addition to a careful history, physical examination, and imaging tests, can help clinicians determine the cause of liver disease in most cases.

The term "liver function tests" is commonly used to refer to a combination of liver biochemical tests, including serum aminotransferases, alkaline phosphatase (AP), and bilirubin. This is a misnomer, because aminotransferases and AP are markers of hepatocyte injury and do not reflect liver synthetic function. Traditionally, liver injury has been characterized as primarily hepatocellular versus cholestatic based on the degree of elevation of aminotransferases compared with AP (**Table 1**). Although such a distinction can help direct initial evaluation, there is often significant overlap in the presentation of various liver diseases, which often have a mixed pattern.[1] It is

Division of Gastroenterology and Hepatology, The Johns Hopkins Hospital, 1830 East Monument Street, Suite 428, Baltimore, MD 21287, USA
* Corresponding author.
E-mail address: salqaht1@jhmi.edu

Med Clin N Am 98 (2014) 1–16
http://dx.doi.org/10.1016/j.mcna.2013.09.005
0025-7125/14/$ – see front matter © 2014 Elsevier Inc. All rights reserved.

Table 1		
Categorization of liver diseases by pattern of elevation of liver enzymes		
Liver Disease Category	**Aminotransferases**	**Alkaline Phosphatase**
Hepatocellular	↑↑	↑
Cholestatic	↑	↑↑

useful to classify liver biochemical tests into the following categories[2]: (1) markers of hepatocellular injury (aminotransferases and AP); (2) tests of liver metabolism (total bilirubin); (3) tests of liver synthetic function (serum albumin and prothrombin time [PT]); and (4) tests for fibrosis in the liver (hyaluronate, type IV collagen, procollagen III, laminin, FibroTest [BioPredictive, Paris, France], and FibroScan [Echosens, Paris, France]).

Furthermore, when evaluating patients with abnormal liver enzyme or function tests, it is helpful to define the liver injury as acute versus chronic. Liver disease is considered chronic if the abnormalities in liver enzyme tests or function persist for more than 6 months.

MARKERS OF HEPATOCELLULAR INJURY

The liver contains a multitude of enzymes in high concentration, some of which are present in the serum in very low concentrations. Injury to the hepatocyte membrane leads to leakage of these enzymes into the serum, which results in increased serum concentrations within a few hours after liver injury. Serum enzymes tests can be categorized into two groups[2]: enzymes whose elevation reflects generalized damage to hepatocytes (aminotransferases); and enzymes whose elevation primarily reflects cholestasis (AP, γ-glutamyltransferase [GGT], 5′ nucleotidase [5′-NT]).

Aminotransferases

The aminotransferases (previously called transaminases) are located in hepatocytes and are sensitive indicators of hepatocyte injury. They are useful in detecting acute hepatocellular diseases, such as hepatitis.[2] They consist of aspartate aminotransferase (AST) and alanine aminotransferase (ALT). Aminotransferases catalyze the transfer of the α-amino groups from aspartate or alanine to the α-keto group of ketoglutaric acid, forming oxaloacetic acid and pyruvic acid, respectively. The enzymatic reduction of oxaloacetic acid and pyruvic acid to malate and lactate, respectively, is coupled to the oxidation of the reduced form of nicotinamide dinucleotide to nicotinamide dinucleotide. Because only nicotinamide dinucleotide absorbs light at 340 nm, this reaction can be followed spectrophotometrically by the loss of absorptivity at 340 nm, and provides an accurate method to assay aminotransferase activity.[3]

AST and ALT are present in the serum at low concentrations, usually less than 30 to 40 IU/L.[4] The normal range varies among clinical laboratories, based on measurements in specific populations. Several factors have been shown to influence ALT activity, such as gender and obesity.[5] Men tend to have a higher serum ALT activity compared with women.

ALT is found in highest concentration in hepatocytes and in very low concentrations in any other tissues. In contrast, AST is found in many other tissues including muscle (cardiac, skeletal, and smooth muscle); kidney; and brain.[2] Thus, ALT is a more specific marker for liver injury. A ratio of AST/ALT greater than five, especially if ALT is normal or slightly elevated, is suggestive of injury to extrahepatic tissues, such as skeletal muscle in the case of rhabdomyolysis or strenuous exercise.

AST is present in the cytoplasm and mitochondria, whereas ALT is only present in the cytoplasm (**Fig. 1**). About 80% of AST activity in the liver is derived from the mitochondrial isoenzyme, whereas most serum AST activity is derived from the cytosolic isoenzyme in healthy persons.[2] Processes leading to necrosis of hepatocytes or damage to the hepatocyte cell membrane with increased permeability result in release of AST and ALT into the blood.[6]

Assessing the pattern and degree of elevation in liver enzymes can help elucidate the cause of liver injury and direct subsequent diagnostic testing and management. Any type of liver cell injury can cause moderate elevations in serum aminotransferase levels. Levels up to 300 IU/L are nonspecific and can be seen in any type of liver disorder.[7] Massive elevations with aminotransferase levels greater than 1000 IU/L are almost exclusively seen in disorders associated with extensive hepatocellular injury, most commonly caused by (1) toxin- or drug-induced liver injury, (2) acute ischemic liver injury, or (3) acute viral hepatitis. Severe autoimmune hepatitis or Wilson disease may also cause markedly elevated aminotransferases.

ALT is present in highest concentration in periportal hepatocytes (Zone 1) and in lowest concentration in hepatocytes surrounding the central vein (Zone 3). AST, however, is present in hepatocytes at more constant levels (**Fig. 2**). Hepatocytes around the central vein have the lowest oxygen concentration and thus are more prone to damage in the setting of acute hepatic ischemia that can occur as the result of acute hypotension or severe cardiac disease. The ensuing centrilobular necrosis results in a rapid rise in aminotransferases, with AST value greater than ALT in the initial days of hepatic injury.

After there is no further injury to hepatocytes, the rate of decline of AST and ALT depends on their rate of clearance from the circulation. AST and ALT are catabolized by the liver, primarily by cells in the reticuloendothethlial system. The plasma half-life of AST and ALT are 17 ± 5 hours and 47 ± 10 hours, respectively.[2] Thus, AST declines more rapidly than ALT, and ALT may be higher than AST in the recovery phase of injury.

Biliary obstruction, such as that caused by a common bile duct stone causing an acute increase in intrabiliary pressure, may also lead to an acute, transient elevation in aminotransferases.

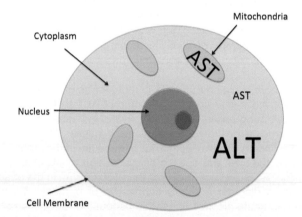

Fig. 1. Location of AST and ALT in hepatocyte. ALT is only present in the cytoplasm, whereas AST is present in both the cytoplasm and mitochondria. Eighty percent of AST activity in the liver is derived from the mitochondrial isoenzyme.

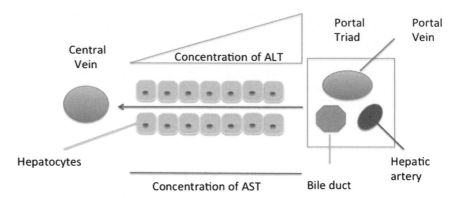

Fig. 2. Concentration of AST and ALT according to location of hepatocytes in portal triad.

A wide variety of disorders can cause chronic elevation in serum transaminases. Nonhepatic causes include thyroid diseases, celiac sprue, anorexia nervosa, Addison disease, and muscle diseases.[3] The most common hepatic causes of chronically elevated liver enzymes are chronic viral hepatitis (hepatitis C and B); alcoholic liver disease; nonalcoholic fatty liver disease; and drugs. Drugs that can cause elevated aminotransferase levels include antituberculosis drugs, such as isoniazid; antifungals, such as azole drugs; and antiepileptic drugs. Other causes of chronic hepatitis include (1) autoimmune hepatitis, which is most commonly seen in women and is associated with other autoimmune diseases; (2) inherited metabolic liver disease, such as hereditary hemochromatosis, Wilson disease, and α_1-antitrypsin deficiency; and (3) infiltrative disorders, such as granulomatous liver diseases.

Aminotransferases levels are typically less than 400 IU/L in alcoholic liver disease. An AST/ALT ratio of greater than two suggests alcoholic liver disease, whereas a ratio greater than three is strongly suggestive.[8] Low AST activity is secondary to a deficiency of pyridoxal 5'-phosphate, which is common in alcoholics.[9] Furthermore, alcohol primarily damages mitochondria, which results in the release of AST into the serum. Elevation in aminotransferase levels to greater than 1000 IU/mL is almost never caused by alcoholic liver disease alone and suggests the presence of a concomitant process, such as drug-induced liver injury or viral hepatitis. Chronic alcoholic use leads to induction of the hepatic cytochrome CYP2E1, which converts acetaminophen to the highly toxic intermediate, N-acetyl-p-benzoquinoneimine. Thus, patients who drink alcohol on a chronic basis are at increased risk of developing acetaminophen hepatotoxicity when consuming acetaminophen, even at doses less than 4 g/day.

Although ALT is more elevated than AST in most forms of chronic liver disease with the exception of alcoholic liver disease, the ratio of AST to ALT changes as fibrosis develops. As fibrosis progresses, the AST/ALT ratio increases and becomes greater than one after cirrhosis has developed in most cases. The platelet count also decreases with advancing fibrosis and cirrhosis, because of the reduction of thrombopoetin synthesis by the liver and splenic sequestration of platelets in the setting of portal hypertension. A platelet count of less than 150,000/μL in the absence of an underlying hematologic disorder is highly suggestive of cirrhosis. Thrombocytopenia may also be seen in acute alcoholic hepatitis because of bone marrow suppression from alcohol toxicity.

Tables 2 and **3** summarize the causes of acute and chronic elevations in aminotransferase levels, their pattern of AST and ALT elevation, and additional diagnostic

Table 2
Hepatic causes of acute elevation in aminotransferase levels and their patterns of liver enzyme injury

Disease	Aminotransferase Levels	Diagnostic Tests	Clinical Clues
Drug- or toxin-induced liver injury			
Acetaminophen	Often >500 IU/L	Acetaminophen level	History of ingestion
Amanita phalloides poisoning	AST > ALT	—	Wild mushroom ingestion
Acute viral hepatitis			
HAV	Often >500 IU/L	Anti-HAV IgM	Risk factors
HBV	ALT > AST	HBsAg, HBV DNA, anti-HBc	
HCV (rare)	—	HCV RNA, anti-HCV	
HDV (in setting of HBV coinfection)	—	Anti-HDV	
HEV	—	HEV IgM	
HSV	—	HSV IgM	
EBV	—	EBV IgM, EBV DNA	
CMV	—	CMV IgM, CMV DNA	
VZV	—	VZV IgM	
Parvovirus B19	—	Parvovirus B19 IgM	
Ischemic hepatitis	Often >500 IU/L AST > ALT	—	Recent hypotension
Alcoholic hepatitis	<400 IU/L	—	History of excess alcohol consumption
	AST: ALT >2		Disproportionate elevation in total bilirubin
Acute biliary obstruction	May be up to 1000 IU/L	Imaging (eg, ultrasound)	Acute onset of right upper quadrant pain
	ALT > AST	—	History of cholelithiasis

Abbreviations: ALT, alanine aminotransferase; AST, aspartate aminotransferase; CMV, cytomegalovirus; EBV, Epstein-Barr virus; HAV, hepatitis A; HBsAg, hepatitis B surface antigen; HBV, hepatitis B virus; HCV, hepatitis C virus; HDV, hepatitis D virus; HEV, hepatitis E virus; HSV, herpes simplex virus; VZV, varicella zoster virus.

testing indicated. An algorithm for the work-up of patients who present with a hepatocellular pattern of liver injury is outlined in **Fig. 3**.

Cholestasis

Cholestasis refers to the pathologic condition in which there is impairment in the liver's ability to secrete bile. Disorders that predominantly affect the biliary system are referred to as cholestatic diseases. They may affect the intrahepatic or extrahepatic bile ducts, or both. In such disorders, the elevation in AP is the predominant feature.

Alkaline phosphatase

AP refers to a group of zinc metalloenzymes that catalyze the hydrolysis of several organic phosphate esters at a neutral pH.[3] APs are found in the canalicular membrane

Table 3
Hepatic causes of chronic elevation in aminotransferase levels and their patterns of liver enzyme injury

Disease	Aminotransferase Levels	Diagnostic Tests	Clinical Clues
Chronic viral hepatitis			
HCV HBV HDV (in setting of HBV coinfection)	<500 IU/L ALT > ALT —	Anti-HCV, HCV RNA HBsAg, HBV DNA Anti-HDV	Risk factors
Alcoholic liver disease	<400 IU/L AST: ALT >2	—	History of excess alcohol consumption
Nonalcoholic fatty liver disease	<300 IU/L ALT > AST	—	History of obesity, diabetes, hyperlipidemia
Drug-induced liver injury	Up to 2000 IU/mL ALT > AST	Improvement after drug discontinuation	Inciting medication
Autoimmune hepatitis	Up to 2000 IU/L ALT > AST	ANA, antismooth muscle antibody IgG levels	Usually women, 30–50 y of age Presence of other autoimmune diseases
Hereditary hemochromatosis	<200 IU/L ALT > AST	Ferritin, iron saturation, HFE gene testing	Family history
Wilson disease	Up to 2000 IU/L ALT > AST	Serum ceruloplasmin 24 h urinary copper collection Slit-lamp examination	Age <40 y Low serum AP —
α_1-antitrypsin deficiency	<100 IU/L	Serum α_1-antitrypsin level	Family history Presence of lung disease at young age
Infiltrative liver disease	<500 IU/L ALT > AST	Imaging Liver biopsy	—
Cirrhosis of any cause	<300 IU/L AST > ALT	—	Platelet count <150,000/μL Signs of portal hypertension

Abbreviations: ALT, alanine aminotransferase; AP, alkaline phosphatase; AST, aspartate aminotransferase; HBsAg, hepatitis B surface antigen; HBV, hepatitis B virus; HCV, hepatitis C virus; HDV, hepatitis D virus; HFE.

of hepatocytes, the membrane of bone osteoblasts, the brush border of small intestinal mucosal cells, the proximal convoluted tubules of the kidney, the placenta, and white blood cells.[2] Most AP in the serum is derived from the liver, bone, and intestine. Individuals with blood type O and B have been shown to have an elevation in serum AP after consumption of a fatty meal.[10] The level of serum AP also varies by age. Individuals older than the age of 60 were found to have higher serum AP levels compared with younger adults.[11] Woman in the third trimester of pregnancy can have elevated serum AP levels because of influx from the placenta.

The first step in the evaluation of an elevated serum AP level in asymptomatic patients is to determine the origin of the elevation. The most widely available and accepted approach is to measure the activity of serum GGT or 5′-NT, liver enzymes that are released in parallel to liver AP.[7] The most precise method to determine the

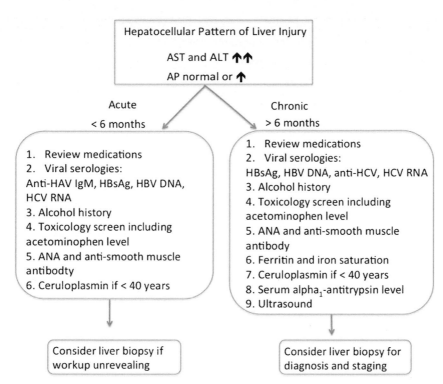

Fig. 3. Algorithm for evaluation of patients with hepatocellular pattern of liver injury. ANA, antinuclear antibodies; HAV, hepatitis A virus; HBsAG, hepatitis B surface antigen; HBV, hepatitis B virus; HCV, hepatitis C virus.

source of AP is to fractionate AP isoenzymes by electrophoresis; however, this is not widely available in most laboratories.

Elevation in serum AP occurs when the hepatocyte canalicular membrane is disrupted, causing translocation from the canalicular membrane to the basolateral (ie, sinusoidal) surface of the hepatocyte and leakage into serum. The mechanism of the increase in AP is thought to be caused by the enhanced translation of messenger RNA (mRNA) of AP in hepatocytes, rather than the failure to excrete AP.[2] This seems to be mediated by the action of bile acids, which induce synthesis of the enzyme and may cause leakage into serum. Hence, in the setting of acute obstruction of the biliary tree caused by gallstones, serum AP may initially be normal as de novo synthesis is required, whereas marked elevation in aminotransferases may be seen.

Hepatocellular disease can lead to an increase in serum AP, which is generally less than three times the upper limit of normal. Thus, moderate elevations in AP are nonspecific and can be seen in viral hepatitis, chronic hepatitis, cirrhosis, congestive heart failure, and infiltrative diseases of the liver.

The pattern of liver injury can be characterized based on the ratio (R) of the serum ALT to AP (both expressed as multiples of the upper limit of normal): an R ratio of less than two indicating cholestatic, greater than five hepatocellular, and two to five as mixed cholestatic-hepatocellular injury.

The most common causes of cholestasis are listed in **Table 4**. Intrahepatic cholestasis is most commonly caused by medications, including certain antibiotics, antiepileptic drugs, and anabolic steroids. It can also be caused by sepsis or total parenteral

Table 4
Common causes of intrahepatic and extrahepatic cholestasis

Disease	Diagnostic Tests	Clinical Clues
Intrahepatic causes		
Primary biliary cirrhosis	Antimitochondrial antibody	Usually middle-aged women Presentation with fatigue or pruritus
Primary sclerosing cholangitis	MRCP or ERCP	Presence of ulcerative colitis
Infiltrative disorders	Imaging	History of tuberculosis, sarcoidosis, amyloidosis, or malignancy
	Liver biopsy	Presentation with weight loss
Medication-induced injury	Improvement after medication discontinuation	Inciting medication
Sepsis	—	History of recent/current infection
TPN	—	TPN use
Extrahepatic causes		
Choledocholithiasis	Ultrasound ERCP or MRCP	History of biliary colic Acute onset of right upper quadrant pain, fever, or jaundice
Primary sclerosing cholangitis	ERCP	Presence of ulcerative colitis
Malignancy		
Pancreatic cancer Cholangiocarcinoma	Imaging (computed tomography or magnetic resonance imaging)	Presentation with jaundice and weight loss

Abbreviations: ERCP, endoscopic retrograde cholangiopancreatography; MRCP, magnetic resonance cholangiopancreatography; TNP, total parenteral nutrition.

nutrition. Several diseases cause injury to the small intrahepatic bile ducts, including primary biliary cirrhosis, primary or secondary sclerosing cholangitis, and infiltrative disorders. Infiltrative disorders of the liver, such as sarcoidosis, tuberculosis, lymphoma, amyloidosis, and metastatic disease to the liver are commonly associated with elevated alkaline phosphatase. Other causes are chronic liver allograft rejection (which leads to ductopenia) and infectious hepatobiliary disorders in patients with AIDS, such as cytomegalovirus or cryptosporidial infection (AIDS cholangioathy).

Causes of extrahepatic obstruction include benign and malignant conditions. Benign causes include choledocholithiasis and primary or secondary cholangitis, which may affect both the intrahepatic and extrahepatic biliary tree. Malignant causes include cholangiocarcinoma, pancreatic, and ampullary cancers.

Imaging of the liver with ultrasonography is indicated in the initial assessment of patients with a predominantly cholestatic pattern of liver enzyme injury to assess for the presence of biliary ductal dilatation. Dilated bile ducts suggest the presence of biliary obstruction and warrants further evaluation with additional imaging (magnetic resonance imaging, magnetic resonance cholangiopancreatography) or endoscopic retrograde cholangiopancreatography for diagnostic and possible therapeutic purposes.

Low levels of AP can present in patients with fulminant Wilson disease and is associated with hemolytic anemia.

γ-glutamyltransferase

GGT is an enzyme that catalyzes the transfer of the γ-glutamyl group of peptides, such as glutathione to other peptides or amino acids. GGT is present in the cell membranes of many tissues including the proximal renal tubule, liver, pancreas, intestine, and spleen.[3] In the liver, GGT is located primarily on biliary epithelial cells and on the apical membrane of hepatocytes. The predominant source of serum GGT is the liver. Entry of GGT into the serum may occur by solubilization and release of membrane-bound GGT or the death of biliary epithelial cells.[12]

Serum GGT is a sensitive indicator of the presence of injury to the bile ducts or liver. However, its use is limited by its lack of specificity, because many nonhepatic disorders can lead to elevation, including diabetes, hyperthyroidism, chronic obstructive pulmonary disease, and renal failure.[13] Alcohol abuse and certain medications, such as barbiturates or phenytoin, lead to induction of hepatic microsomal GGT.[14] The main clinical use of GGT is to confirm the hepatic origin of elevated AP levels, because GGT is not elevated in patients with bone disease.

5′ nucleotidase

5′-NT catalyzes the hydrolysis of nucleotides, such as adenosine 5′-phosphate and inosine 5′-phosphate, resulting in the release of free inorganic phosphate, which is most commonly measured by assays of its activity. 5′-NT is found in the liver, intestine, brain, heart, blood vessels, and pancreas.[2] In the liver, it is found bound to the canalicular and sinusoidal membrane of hepatocytes. Its activity parallels that of AP, which is likely a reflection of their similar location in the hepatocyte.[15] Most studies show that 5′-NT and AP have equal clinical use in the detection of hepatobiliary disease.[2] Like GGT, its clinical value lies in its ability to determine the origin of elevated serum AP levels, because its elevation in this setting strongly suggests a hepatic origin. The algorithm for the evaluating patients with a predominant elevation in AP is summarized in **Fig. 4**.

TESTS OF LIVER METABOLISM: TOTAL BILIRUBIN

Bilirubin is a naturally occurring pigment derived from the breakdown of heme-containing proteins. Most of the 250 to 300 mg of bilirubin produced each day is derived from the breakdown of hemoglobin in senescent red blood cells.[16] The remainder is derived from the premature destruction of erythroid cells in the bone marrow and from the turnover of heme-containing proteins in tissues in the body.[17] The liver has a high concentration of heme-containing proteins with high turnover rates, such as the cytochrome P-450 enzymes.

The formation of bilirubin occurs primarily in reticuloendothelial cells in the liver and spleen. The first step consists of the oxidation of heme by heme oxygenase to form biliverdin. The second reaction is the reduction of biliverdin by biliverdin reductase to form bilirubin. Unconjugated bilirubin is lipid-soluble and insoluble in water. Thus, to be transported in blood, unconjugated bilirubin must be bound to albumin, which occurs in a reversible, noncovalent fashion. Unconjugated bilirubin is thus not filtered by the kidney because it is always bound to albumin in the serum. Bilirubin is then transported to the liver, where it is taken up by hepatocytes by carrier-mediated membrane transport. In the hepatocyte, it is bound to glutathione-S-transferases. Bilirubin is then conjugated by a family of enzymes called uridine diphospho-glucuronosyltransferase (UDP-glucuronosyltransferase). Conjugated bilirubin is water-soluble and thus may be excreted by the kidney. Conjugated bilirubin is transported across the canalicular membrane into bile by active transport against a concentration using ATP. This is the rate-limiting step in bilirubin excretion.[2]

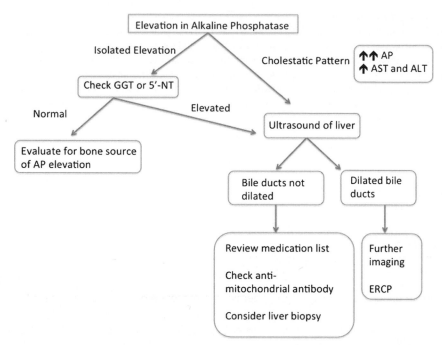

Fig. 4. Algorithm for evaluation of patients with elevated alkaline phosphatase. ERCP, endoscopic retrograde cholangiopancreatography.

The terms direct and indirect bilirubin originated from the van den Bergh method of measuring bilirubin concentration.[18] In the assay, bilirubin reacts with diazotized sulfanilic acid and divides into two dipyrrl azopigments that absorb light maximally at 540 nm. The direct fraction reacts with diazotized sulfanilic acid in 1 minute in the absence of alcohol, and provides an estimate of the concentration of conjugated bilirubin in the serum. The total serum bilirubin concentration is then ascertained by the addition of alcohol and determination of the amount that reacts in 30 minutes. The indirect fraction is thus calculated as the difference between the total and direct bilirubin concentrations. Normal total serum bilirubin concentration is less than 1 mg/dL using the van den Bergh method of bilirubin measurement. The direct fraction comprises as much as 30% or 0.3 mg/dL of the total.

Newer techniques for the measurement of serum bilirubin use high-performance liquid chromatography. These techniques have revealed that almost all of serum bilirubin in healthy persons is unconjugated. Furthermore, it seems that there is a fraction of conjugated bilirubin that is covalently bound to albumin.[19] This fraction increases in patients with cholestasis and hepatobiliary disorders, when the excretion of conjugated bilirubin is impaired, resulting in increased serum concentration of conjugated bilirubin. This explains the prolonged elevation in bilirubin seen in patients recovering from hepatobiliary injury, because the clearance rate of bilirubin bound to albumin from serum is determined by long half-life of albumin (about 21 days) and not the shorter half-life of bilirubin (about 4 hours).[19] This also explains why bilirubinuria is not present in some patients with conjugated hyperbilirubinemia during the recovery phase of their illness.

The concentration of bilirubin in the serum is determined by the balance between bilirubin production and clearance by hepatocytes. Thus, elevated serum bilirubin levels may be caused by (1) excessive bilirubin production, which occurs in states of increased red blood cell turnover, such as hemolytic anemias or hematoma resorption; (2) impaired uptake, conjugation, or excretion of bilirubin; and (3) release of unconjugated or conjugated bilirubin from injured hepatocytes or bile ducts.[7]

The presence of unconjugated hyperbilirubinemia (defined as direct bilirubin fraction <20%) is rarely caused by liver disease. It is primarily seen in hemolytic disorders, such as sickle cell disease or hereditary spherocytosis, or in setting of hematoma resorption. In general, the total serum bilirubin is less than 5 mg/dL in such cases. If hemolysis is ruled out, the most likely cause of mild elevation in indirect bilirubin in an otherwise asymptomatic patient is Gilbert syndrome. This is the result of a genetic defect leading to a mild decrease in the activity of UDP-glucuronosyltransferase. Total bilirubin is usually in the range of 2 to 4 mg/dL. Levels increase during times of fasting or stress. No further evaluation is indicated if Gilbert disease is suspected, because there are no clinical sequelae. Crigler-Najjar syndrome type 1 is a rare, autosomal-recessive disorder that results from near complete absence of UDP-glucuronosyltransferase and leads to severe unconjugated hyperbilirubinemia and kernicterus in newborns. Crigler-Najjar syndrome type 2 results from a milder form of UDP-glucuronosyltransferase deficiency, and patients are generally asymptomatic.

Unlike unconjugated hyperbilirubinemia, the presence of conjugated hyperbilirubinemia (and hence hyperbilirubinuria) almost always signifies the existence of liver disease. Both hepatocellular and cholestatic liver injury may lead to elevated serum bilirubin levels.[20,21]

There are rare inherited disorders in which bilirubin excretion into the bile is impaired, resulting in conjugated hyperbilirubinemia, namely Rotor syndrome and Dubin-Johnson syndrome. Both conditions have a benign clinical course. The algorithm for the evaluation of patients with hyperbilirubinemia is summarized in **Fig. 5**.

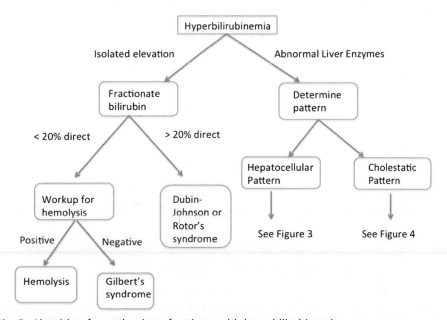

Fig. 5. Algorithm for evaluation of patients with hyperbilirubinemia.

TESTS OF LIVER SYNTHETIC FUNCTION

The liver is the exclusive site of synthesis of albumin and most coagulation factors. Thus, serum albumin and PT serve as true tests of hepatic synthetic function.

Serum albumin has a long half-life of about 21 days. About 4% is degraded per day. Because of its long half-life, serum albumin levels may not be affected in acute liver disease, such as acute viral hepatitis or drug-induced liver injury. In cirrhosis or chronic liver disease, low serum albumin may be a sign of advanced liver disease. However, low serum albumin is not specific for liver disease, and may occur in other conditions, such as malnutrition, infections, nephrotic syndrome, or protein-losing enteropathy.[7]

PT/international normalized ratio (INR) measures the activity of coagulation factors II, V, VII, and X, which are all synthesized in the liver and dependent on vitamin K for synthesis. Coagulation factors have a much shorter half-life than albumin. Thus, PT/INR is the best measure of liver synthetic function in the acute setting. Prolongation of the PT to more than 5 seconds above the control value (INR>1.5) is a poor prognostic sign in liver disease, and an important factor in priority of liver transplantation in model of end-stage liver disease score.

Elevation in PT/INR is also a predictor of high mortality in patients with acute alcoholic hepatitis. Vitamin K deficiency also causes prolongation in PT, and is associated with poor nutrition, malabsorption, and severe cholestasis with inability to absorb fat-soluble vitamins. Administration of parental vitamin K can help distinguish vitamin K deficiency from hepatocyte dysfunction, because it results in the correction of PT in the case of vitamin K deficiency but not liver dysfunction.[2] **Table 5** summarizes the general pattern of liver enzymes and liver function tests seen in the different categories of hepatobiliary disease.

NONINVASIVE MARKERS OF FIBROSIS

Noninvasive tests of hepatic fibrosis have been studied extensively in many clinical trials. Most studies of serologic markers and radiologic tests have looked at the use of these tests for staging of fibrosis in patients with chronic liver disease.[22–24]

There are two general categories of noninvasive tests for fibrosis: serologic panels of tests and radiologic tests. These include indicators of cytolysis (AST, ALT); cholestasis (GGT, bilirubin); hepatocellular synthetic function (INR, cholesterol, ApoA1, haptoglobin, N-glycans); and hypersplenism caused by portal hypertension (ie, platelet count). The most studied panels are the AST to platelet ratio, FibroTest/FibroSure (Labcorp, Burlington, USA), Hepascore (Quest Diagnostics, USA), and FibroSpect (Prometheus Alb Inc., USA).

Radiologic methods for staging hepatic fibrosis are emerging as promising tools. The methods include ultrasound-based transient elastography and magnetic resonance elastography. Ultrasound-based transient elastography using a probe (FibroScan) is the most studied radiologic method for staging hepatic fibrosis. Fibroscan was approved by Food and Drug Administration in April 2013. Using FibroScan in United States becoming more popular as a reliable noninvasive method of assessing liver fibrosis.

APPROACH TO PATIENT EVALUATION AND DIAGNOSIS

The first step in evaluating patients found to have liver enzyme abnormalities is to take a careful and thorough medical history. Risk factors for viral hepatitis including travel history, sexual practices, illicit drug use, acquisition of tattoos, body

Table 5
Patterns of liver enzymes and liver function tests in various hepatobiliary diseases

Hepatobiliary Disorder	Aminotransferases	Alkaline Phosphatase	Bilirubin	Albumin	Prothrombin Time
Hepatocellular					
Acute Toxin/drug Viral Ischemic	↑↑↑ (>500 IU/mL)	Normal or ↑ to <3 times normal	↑	Normal	Usually normal ↑ to >5 seconds above control value portends poor prognosis
Chronic	↑↑ (<300 IU/mL)	Normal or ↑ to <3 times normal	Normal to ↑	Normal or ↓	Often ↑, will not correct with parenteral vitamin K administration
Cholestatic					
Acute	Normal to ↑↑↑	Normal to ↑	Normal to ↑	Normal	Normal
Chronic	Normal to ↑↑	↑↑↑ to >4 times normal	↑	Normal or ↓	Normal or ↑, will correct with vitamin K administration
Infiltrative	Normal to ↑	↑↑↑ to >4 times normal	Normal	Normal	Normal

piercings, occupational exposure, and history of blood transfusions before 1990 should be ascertained. The presence of prodromal symptoms, such as nausea, vomiting, abdominal pain, anorexia, malaise, fevers, or chills suggestive of acute viral hepatitis, should be elicited. A history of significant weight loss raises the possibility of malignancy. Inquiry into the development of jaundice, dark urine, or light stools is important. The acute onset of right upper quadrant pain, fever, or jaundice suggests biliary obstruction caused by gallstones. History of pruritus suggests cholestasis.

Clinicians should inquire about the consumption of alcohol, including frequency, quantity, and duration. A history of obesity, diabetes mellitus, or hyperlipidemia in the absence of significant alcohol consumption suggests the possibility of nonalcoholic fatty liver disease. Meticulous review of the patient's medication list and inquiry into the use of any over-the-counter or herbal medications or nutritional supplements should be performed. A history of inflammatory bowel disease raises the possibility of primary sclerosing cholangitis. Finally, a family history of liver disease is important because it suggests possible inherited liver disorders.

The physical examination is also an important diagnostic tool in the assessment of patients with suspected liver disease. The presence of scleral icterus or jaundice should be assessed. Hepatomegaly may be present in acute viral hepatitis, alcoholic hepatitis, infiltrative liver disorders, or severe congestive hepatopathy caused by heart failure. Temporal wasting and cachexia suggest advanced liver disease or malignancy. Clinicians should assess for stigmata of chronic liver disease, including spider angiomas, palmar erythema, and gynecomastia. Splenomegaly and caput medusa suggests the presence of portal hypertension. Signs of decompensated cirrhosis include the presence of ascites, jaundice, or asterixis/encephalopathy.

If an asymptomatic patient is found to have a first-time elevation in liver enzymes, it is reasonable to observe the patient if (1) no risk factors for liver diseases are identified; (2) the elevation in liver enzymes is mild (ie, less than twice the upper limit of normal); and (3) liver synthetic function is preserved.[4] Repeat testing should be performed within 3 months. If the liver enzymes remain elevated at 3 months, work-up for liver disease should be initiated based on the pattern of liver enzyme elevation as detailed previously.

Liver biopsy remains the gold standard for the grading of inflammation and staging of fibrosis in chronic liver disease, and plays an important role in determining the need for treatment and assessing response to therapy.

SUMMARY

The routine use of serum biochemical tests allows for the detection of acute and chronic liver injury before the onset of symptoms. These tests consist of markers of hepatocellular injury (aminotransferases and APs); tests of liver metabolism (total bilirubin); and tests of liver synthetic function (serum albumin and PT). Noninvasive tests for assessment of liver fibrosis are promising tools for diagnosis and prognosis of patients with chronic liver disease. A comprehensive history, physical examination, and assessment of pattern of liver injury with additional laboratory and imaging testing establish the cause of hepatobiliary disease in most cases.

ACKNOWLEDGMENTS

This work was supported by research grant from HRH Meshal Bin Abdulah Al Saud Foundation.

REFERENCES

1. Green RM, Flamm S. AGA technical review on the evaluation of liver chemistry tests. Gastroenterology 2002;123(4):1367–84.
2. Franklin Herlong FH, Mitchell MC. Laboratory tests. In: Maddrey WC, Schiff ER, Sorrell MF, editors. Schiff's diseases of the liver. Wiley-Blackwell; 2012. p. 17–43.
3. Mukherjee S, Gollan JL. Assessment of liver function. In: Lok AS, Dooley JS, Burroughs AK, et al, editors. Sherlock's diseases of the liver and biliary system. Wiley-Blackwell; 2011. p. 20–35.
4. Pratt DS, Kaplan MM. Evaluation of abnormal liver-enzyme results in asymptomatic patients. N Engl J Med 2000;342(17):1266–71.
5. Piton A, et al. Factors associated with serum alanine transaminase activity in healthy subjects: consequences for the definition of normal values, for selection of blood donors, and for patients with chronic hepatitis C. MULTIVIRC Group. Hepatology 1998;27(5):1213–9.
6. Floch MH, Floch NR, Kowdley KV, et al. Netter's gastroenterology. 1st edition. Carlstadt (NJ): Icon Learning Systems; 2005. p. 900.
7. Longo DL, et al. Harrison's gastroenterology and hepatology. New York: McGraw-Hill Medical; 2010. p. 738.
8. Cohen JA, Kaplan MM. The SGOT/SGPT ratio–an indicator of alcoholic liver disease. Dig Dis Sci 1979;24(11):835–8.
9. Diehl AM, et al. Relationship between pyridoxal 5'-phosphate deficiency and aminotransferase levels in alcoholic hepatitis. Gastroenterology 1984;86(4):632–6.
10. Bamford KF, et al. Serum-alkaline-phosphatase and the ABO blood-groups. Lancet 1965;1(7384):530–1.
11. Heino AE, Jokipii SG. Serum alkaline phosphatase levels in the aged. Ann Med Intern Fenn 1962;51:105–9.
12. Sotil EU, Jensen DM. Serum enzymes associated with cholestasis. Clin Liver Dis 2004;8(1):41–54.
13. Goldberg DM, Martin JV. Role of gamma-glutamyl transpeptidase activity in the diagnosis of hepatobiliary disease. Digestion 1975;12(4–6):232–46.
14. Rollason JG, Pincherle G, Robinson D. Serum gamma glutamyl transpeptidase in relation to alcohol consumption. Clin Chim Acta 1972;39(1):75–80.
15. Righetti A, Kaplan MM. Disparate responses of serum and hepatic alkaline phosphatase and 5' nucleotidase to bile duct obstruction in the rat. Gastroenterology 1972;62(5):1034–9.
16. Lester R, Schmid R. Bilirubin metabolism. N Engl J Med 1964;270:779–86.
17. Robinson SH, et al. Early-labeled peak of bile pigment in man. Studies with glycine-14C and delta-aminolevulinic acid-3H. N Engl J Med 1967;277(25):1323–9.
18. Zieve L, et al. Normal and abnormal variations and clinical significance of the one-minute and total serum bilirubin determinations. J Lab Clin Med 1951;38(3):446–69.
19. Weiss JS, et al. The clinical importance of a protein-bound fraction of serum bilirubin in patients with hyperbilirubinemia. N Engl J Med 1983;309(3):147–50.
20. American Gastroenterological Association. American Gastroenterological Association medical position statement: evaluation of liver chemistry tests. Gastroenterology 2002;123(4):1364–6.
21. Polson J, Lee WM, American Association for the Study of Liver. AASLD position paper: the management of acute liver failure. Hepatology 2005;41(5):1179–97.

22. Miyake T, et al. Real-time tissue elastography for evaluation of hepatic fibrosis and portal hypertension in nonalcoholic fatty liver diseases. Hepatology 2012; 56(4):1271–8.
23. Berzigotti A, et al. Non-invasive diagnostic and prognostic evaluation of liver cirrhosis and portal hypertension. Dis Markers 2011;31(3):129–38.
24. Crespo G, Fernández-Varo G, Mariño Z, et al. ARFI, FibroScan, ELF, and their combinations in the assessment of liver fibrosis: a prospective study. J Hepatol 2012;57(2):281.

Removal Notice

Removal Notice to "An Overview of Emerging Therapies for the Treatment of Chronic Hepatitis C"

Med Clin N Am 98 (2014) 17–38

Jawad A. Ilyas[a,b,c], John M. Vierling[a,b,c]

[a]Liver Center, St Luke's Episcopal Hospital, Baylor College of Medicine, 1709 Dryden, Suite 1500, Houston, TX 77030, USA
[b]Department of Medicine, Baylor College of Medicine, 1709 Dryden Street, Suite 500, Houston, TX 77030, USA
[c]Department of Surgery, Baylor College of Medicine, 1709 Dryden Street, Suite 1500, Houston, TX 77030, USA

This article has been removed: please see Elsevier Policy on Article Withdrawal (http://www.elsevier.com/locate/withdrawalpolicy).

This article has been removed at the request of the Publisher.

This article has been removed because it was published without the permission of the authors.

http://dx.doi.org/10.1016/j.mcna.2014.01.001
0025-7125/14/$ – see front matter.

Chronic Hepatitis B Virus Infection

Brian J. McMahon, MD, MACP

KEYWORDS

- Chronic hepatitis B • Natural history • Management

KEY POINTS

- The Centers for Disease Control and Prevention (CDC) recommend that people born in Asia, Africa, or other regions endemic for hepatitis B virus (HBV) should be tested for hepatitis B surface antigen and antibody to hepatitis B surface antigen (anti-HBs), as 2% to 10% will have chronic HBV.
- All people with chronic HBV infection should be followed regularly (every 6 months), as HBV infection can have a complicated course progressing through several phases that can be further complicated by regression back to earlier phases.
- Candidates for antiviral therapy include patients with moderate-to-severe liver disease as determined by elevated alanine aminotransferase and/or liver biopsy and elevated HBV DNA levels above 2000 IU/mL as per evidenced-based practice guidelines.
- Antiviral medications of choice are pegylated interferon, entecavir, or tenofovir in treatment-naïve patients and pegylated interferon or tenofovir in lamivudine-experienced patients.
- All persons undergoing cancer chemotherapy or immunosuppressive therapy should be screened for hepatitis B and given HBV antiviral prophylaxis if chronically infected.

INTRODUCTION

Chronic hepatitis B virus (HBV) is one of the most common chronic infections in the world. An estimated 2 billion people have been infected, and up to 400,000 people worldwide are believed to have chronic HBV.[1] This article discusses the epidemiology, natural history, and clinical management of HBV, but also highlights some special circumstances that are associated with chronic HBV infection.

EPIDEMIOLOGY OF HBV AND SCREENING FOR PATIENTS WITH CHRONIC HBV INFECTION

Prevalence of HBV Worldwide and Whom to Screen for HBV in Developed Countries

In most countries of the world, the prevalence of people with chronic HBV, defined as hepatitis B surface antigen (HBsAg)-positive for at least 6 months, is over 2%. The

Liver Disease and Hepatitis Program, Alaska Native Tribal Health Consortium, 4315 Diplomacy Drive, Anchorage, AK 99508, USA
E-mail address: bmcmahon@anthc.org

Med Clin N Am 98 (2014) 39–54
http://dx.doi.org/10.1016/j.mcna.2013.08.004
0025-7125/14/$ – see front matter
© 2014 Elsevier Inc. All rights reserved.
medical.theclinics.com

prevalence is 8% or more in much of Africa and Asia (**Fig. 1**).[2] In western countries, including the United States and western Europe, the Centers for Disease Control and Prevention (CDC) recommend testing everyone born in Asian-Pacific regions (except Japan), Africa, eastern and southern Europe, Central America except Mexico, and selected indigenous populations in developed countries. In addition, certain other high-risk groups in which the prevalence of HBsAg is above 2% (a level shown to be cost-effective by the CDC), such as household and sexual partners of persons with chronic HBV, men who have sex with men, human immunodeficiency virus (HIV)-infected patients, and institutionalized patients, should be tested.[3] Other high-risk groups should be screened for vaccination, such as people with multiple sexual partners, and intravenous drug uses, understanding that they have a lower risk of chronic HBV. The Hepatitis B Foundation sponsored a panel of experts in primary care and hepatology who developed a very useful algorithm for screening and management of HBV (**Fig. 2**, **Table 1**).[4]

Risk of Developing Chronic HBV After Acute Infection

Table 2 shows the risk of developing chronic HBV after acute HBV infection. Risk is highest in infants whose mothers are HBsAg positive[5] as well as in children infected under 5 years of age through horizontal transmission by open bug bites, cuts, scratches, or impetigo sores.[6] HBV is infectious outside the body on environmental surfaces for at least 7 days and likely much longer, making this the most infectious viral agent in these circumstances.[7]

Natural History of Chronic HBV

Patients with chronic HBV infection can have a complicated course progressing through several phases that can be further complicated by regression back to earlier

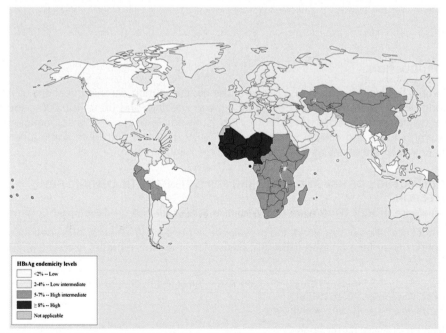

Fig. 1. Global prevalence of chronic hepatitis B infection. (*Courtesy of* Centers for Disease Control and Prevention, Atlanta, GA.)

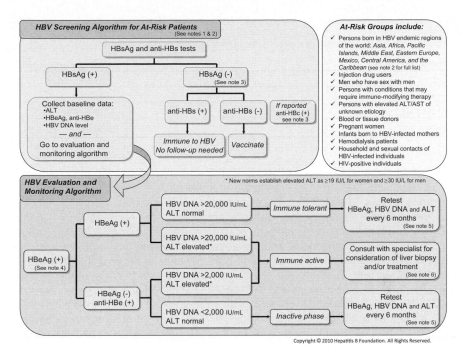

Fig. 2. Hepatitis B foundation algorithm for screening and management of hepatitis B. (*From* McHugh JA, Cullison S, Apuzzio J, et al. Chronic hepatitis B infection: a workshop consensus statement and algorithm. J Fam Pract 2011;60(9):E1–8; with permission. Copyright © 2011 Quadrant Health Com Inc.)

Table 1	
High-risk persons who should be screened for HBV	
Contacts	Household contacts
	Sex partners of persons with chronic HBV
	Clients and staff in institutions for developmentally disabled
	Correctional facility inmates
	Travelers (for >6 mo to countries with high or intermediate prevalence of HBV)
Behavioral	Intravenous drug users
	More than 1 sex partner in previous 6 mo
	Recently acquired sexually transmitted disease (STD), including all clients in STD clinics
	Men who have sex with men
Occupational	Health professionals
	Public safety workers with exposure to blood
Medical	Hemodialysis
	Patients receiving clotting factor concentrates

Data from Weinbaum CM, Mast EE, Ward JW. Recommendations for identification and public health management of persons with chronic hepatitis B virus infection. Hepatology 2009;49(5):S35–44.

Table 2 Age-specific risk of developing chronic HBV infection after exposure	
Age at Exposure	**Risk of Chronic HBV**
Birth	90%
Infancy to 2 y	50%
Infancy to 5 y	25%–30%
Above 5 y	5%–7%

phases.[8] At National Institutes of Health (NIH) workshop, 4 phases of chronic HBV were identified: the immune-tolerant, immune-active, inactive, and HBsAg-clearance phases.[9] **Table 3** details the 4 phases of chronic HBV.

In the immune-tolerant phase, patients are positive for hepatitis B "e" antigen (HBeAg), and their immune systems do not recognize this virus as a foreign invader, which results in high viral loads and no elevation of alanine aminotransferase (ALT) levels or liver inflammation. This phase is primarily seen in patients infected at birth from HBeAg-positive mothers who are usually infected with HBV genotype C, found in eastern and southeast Asian and the Pacific Islands regions as well as northwest Alaska,[10] or certain subtypes of genotype B recombined with genotype C in east Asia. As people in the immune-tolerant phase age, their immune systems begin to recognize this virus and mount a response, resulting in elevation of ALT followed by reduction in the levels of HBV DNA (the immune-active phase) and eventual loss of HBeAg and development of antibody to HBeAg (anti-HBe). People exposed after birth, primarily with genotypes A, B1 and B6, D, E, and F, who develop chronic infection, often skip the immune-tolerant phase and go right into the immune-active phase. These genotypes are most commonly found in Africa, the Middle East, Europe, the Indian subcontinent and southwestern Alaska. Between 65% and 75% of these patients over time will mount a strong immune response and suppress HBV DNA to low levels (below 1000 IU/ml) and have normalization of their ALT levels that is often permanent, the inactive HBV phase. Their risk of developing cirrhosis due to HBV is very low, if indeed at all, and liver fibrosis can slowly reverse and even disappear over time. Some of these patients will eventually lose HBsAg at a rate of 0.5% to 2.0% per year[11–13] and, while they are still at risk for liver cancer, that risk will decrease several fold. Unfortunately, a minority of patients who lose HBeAg can revert back to HBeAg, usually accompanied by an asymptomatic flare of hepatitis, and up to 20% of those who develop anti-HBe can have chronic hepatitis despite HBeAg seroconversion or reactivate their hepatitis when seeming to be in the inactive phase.[14] Thus, patients with chronic HBV need to be followed carefully for life.

The 2 most dreaded complications of chronic HBV are hepatocellular carcinoma (HCC) and end-stage cirrhosis. Prospective population-based studies have shown that 20% to 40% of men and 15% of women with chronic HBV who are infected early in life develop HCC.[15,16] Although the data are not as good for end-stage liver disease or decompensated cirrhosis, it has been estimated that 10% to 15% of patients will die of this complication. Risk factors for developing HCC include male gender, coinfection with HIV, hepatitis C virus (HCV) or hepatitis delta virus (HDV), HBV genotype, HBV DNA of greater than 20,000 IU/mL, and mutation in the basal core promoter region (BCP) of the virus.[10,17] A mutation in the precore (PC) region of the virus was previously thought to be a risk factor, but the only large population-based study that looked at this found the PC mutation was associated with a lower risk of HCC. This was also seen in a population-based nested case–control study from Alaska.[18,19]

Table 3
Four phases of chronic HBV infection

Phase	HBeAg	ALT Level	HBV DNA Level	Liver Histology	Potential Treatment Candidate	Risk of HCC[a] for Patients >40 y
Immune-Tolerant	Positive	Normal	>20,000 IU/mL	Normal	No	+++
ImmuneActive	Positive or Negative	Elevated	>2000 IU/mL	Mild-to-severe inflammation/fibrosis	Yes	+++
Inactive	Negative	Normal	<2000 IU/mL	Improving histology	No	++
HBsAg Clearance	—	Normal	<1000 IU/mL	Improving histology	No	+

[a] Compared with the general US population.

Although BCP and PC are commercially available, as noted previously, PC has not been validated to have value in predicting increased risk for HCC; plus PC is often present in HBeAg-negative patients without HCC, making it difficult to apply to individual patients. Heavy alcohol use, smoking, and exposure to aflatoxin, found in moldy grains and nuts in Africa and Asia, are also risk factors for HCC. High levels of HBV DNA, elevated ALT, and a family history of HCC are also risk factors.[20,21] The risks of HCC and cirrhosis are low in those under 35 years of age, but they rise exponentially in men over 40 and women over 50.[22]

HBV Genotypes

There are at least 8 HBV genotypes that differ by greater than 8% in complete sequence, and many subgenotypes that differ by at least 4%.[10] Disease outcome is strongly influenced by genotype, but, with the exception of interferon therapy, response to treatment is not. This is the opposite what has been found with HCV infection. Genotypes A1, A3, and E are found in Africa and are associated with high rates of HCC, especially in younger men, but not often associated with cirrhosis. Genotype A2 is found in northern Europe. Genotype B has many subtypes but can be divided into pure B (B1 found in Japan and B6 found in the Arctic) and the other subtypes, which have a recombination of a piece of genotype C in the core region of the viral genome. This recombinant B, referred to as Ba for Asia, is associated with greater risk of liver cancer and cirrhosis, whereas B1 and B6, along with A2, are associated with less of a risk of cirrhosis that occurs much later in life. Genotype C is documented to be the most aggressive, with high rates of HCC and cirrhosis starting in the fifth decade of life. It is also associated with a prolonged period of HBeAg seropositivity and higher risk of perinatal transmission than the other genotypes. Genotype D is associated with HBeAg-negative cirrhosis and HCC, although the risk is lower than for C or Ba. Genotype F is associated with high rates of HCC in children in Alaska,[18] and more aggressive disease in the Amazon Basin. Genotype H has not been well studied, and genotype G is usually found in a recombinant form, mostly with genotype A. In the United States, HBV genotype reflects the region where infected patients are from. with genotypes B and C found in Asians and South Pacific Islanders; A1, A3, and E are found in Africa as well as in immigrants born in Africa. HBV genotypes A1, A3, Ba, C, E, and F are associated with higher rates of HCC than other genotypes.[10] However, rates of chronic HBV are low in US-born African Americans and Hispanic persons born in Mexico. Genotypes A and D are found in patients from Europe, the Indian subcontinent and the Middle East. **Fig. 3** displays the geographic distribution of HBV genotypes.

MANAGEMENT OF CHRONIC HBV

The 3 major liver societies, the American Association for the Study of Liver Diseases (AASLD), the European and Asian Pacific Associations for the Liver (EASL and APASL, respectively) have all written evidenc-based practice guidelines for chronic hepatitis B that are updated every 3 to 5 years.[23–25] All 3 guidelines are much more similar than different, and all stress that people with chronic HBV infection must be followed on a regular basis every 3 to 12 months for life depending on disease activity, regardless of what phase of the disease they are in. There is strong evidence that treatment of patients with compensated cirrhosis decreases the risk of HCC, liver failure, and liver-related death from a large randomized trial conducted in Taiwan and several clinic-based case–control trials.[2,26] There is also evidence that treatment of persons with cirrhosis, advanced fibrosis, or moderate fibrosis leads to reversal of fibrosis in

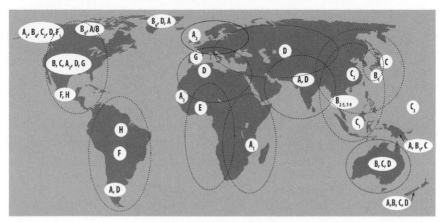

Fig. 3. Worldwide distribution of HBV genotypes and subgenotypes. (*Courtesy of* Centers for Disease Control and Prevention, Atlanta, GA; and *From* Spradling PR, Hu DJ, McMahon BJ. Epidemiology and prevention. In: Thomas H, Zuckerman A, Lok A, et al, editors. Viral Hepatitis: 4th Edition. Hoboken: Wiley-Blackwell; 2014.)

most people, and the actual reversal of cirrhosis after 5 years of viral suppression from treatment in many patients has been shown.[27] HBV cannot be cured for 2 reasons: (1) the virus persists in liver cells for years in a double-stranded closed circular DNA form, and (2) HBV uses a reverse transcriptase to replicate, allowing the virus to integrate pieces of its genome into the DNA of the human host liver cell, thus increasing the susceptible to carcinogenic transformation. In fact, unlike HCV, where the risk of cancer is increased only in those with advanced fibrosis or cirrhosis, HCC can occur in noncirrhotic livers of HBV-infected patients.[28]

Routine Monitoring of Patients with Chronic HBV

When a patient is first identified to have chronic HBV infection, the initial laboratory evaluation should include a full liver panel, complete blood count (CBC), and HBV DNA to categorize the phase of HBV present (see **Fig. 2**).[4] Because chronic HBV infection is life long, patients must be monitored on regular basis indefinitely; every 6 months is a reasonable interval.[23] Those patients in the immune-active phase should be monitored more frequently and those who have been in the inactive phase for several years could be monitored yearly. Liver function tests should performed at 6-month intervals and platelet counts yearly, because a falling platelet count below 150,000 suggests that advanced fibrosis could be present. HBV DNA levels should be done at least whenever ALT levels are elevated and periodically in those with normal ALT levels. A baseline liver ultrasound with a portal flow study can pick up signs of cirrhosis such as the presence of a dense, nodular liver, as well as signs of portal hypertension including reversal of portal blood flow on Doppler study, splenomegaly, varices, and small amounts of ascites not detected on physical examination. In persons without overt signs of liver failure who have laboratory tests suggesting advanced fibrosis and declining synthetic liver function including a platelet count falling below 150,000, a lower than normal albumin or elevated total and direct bilirubin should have a prothrombin time (PT)/INR performed to determine if a coagulopathy is present, which would lead the clinician to start antiviral therapy to prevent liver failure, HCC, or liver related death.

Tests used to assess and monitor progression liver fibrosis may be helpful in a limited number of patients. These include such commercially available tests such as

FibroTest (LabCor, USA), FibroSpect II (Prometheus Laboratories, San Diego, CA), and tests using simple formulas and routine laboratory tests to calculate fibrosis such as APRI (AST to platelet ratio index) and Fib-4 (age, ALT, aspartate aminotransferase [AST] and platelet count). These tests have high specificity (but low sensitivity) in evaluating the amount of fibrosis at the end of their ranges of values, namely in persons with little or no fibrosis and those with advanced fibrosis, but they are not much better than a flip of the coin in those in between.[29,30] For example, the APRI has 90% specificity but only about 50% sensitivity for no or mild fibrosis at scores less than 0.5 and of advanced fibrosis/cirrhosis at scores above 1.5 with little correlation in between. In HCV, a FibroTest score of 0.7 had 98% sensitivity and 76% positive predictive value for detection of bridging fibrosis (F3) or cirrhosis (F4), while a FibroTest less than or equal to 0.3 had 92% sensitivity and 98% negative predictive value. In between these values, however, the test is not helpful.[31]

Fibroscan is a radiologic examination that can be administered by clinicians and has been increasingly studied in the setting of chronic HBV and HCV infections. It recently was licensed in the United States. This machine uses pulses of ultrasound waves shot into the liver to give a reading of the quantity of fibrosis. It is useful in patients with advanced fibrosis, with an area under the curve for accuracy of approximately 0.9.[32] Although it is not as useful in assessing lesser amounts of fibrosis, it can be useful if following patient scores over time. The limitations of Fibroscan include the inability to obtain a reading in obese patients, operator experience, and false-positive readings in persons with flares of HBV and high ALT levels.[33,34] A new probe has been developed that will hopefully be more useful in obese patients.

There has been recent interest in the use of HBsAg levels to determine phase of HBV and predict progression of disease.[35] In general, HBsAg levels are highest in patients in the immune-tolerant phase, and stepwise lower in those in the immune-active and inactive phases, respectively.[36,37] A recent study showed that levels of HBsAg below 1000 IU/mL combined with HBV DNA levels below 2000 IU/mL can predict that patients in the inactive phase will remain there with a high level of accuracy.[36] The clinical usefulness of HBsAg levels in practice remains to be sorted out by future studies.

Use of Liver Biopsy

Current evidenced-based practice guidelines by the 3 major liver societies all recommend that people with an elevated ALT level and evidence of active liver inflammation, who can be shown to have moderate-to-severe inflammation or fibrosis, are candidates for antiviral therapy.[23–25] Liver biopsy will not be needed in those in whom evidence of advanced fibrosis can be demonstrated by noninvasive methods, including any of the following: liver ultrasound, Fibroscan, clinical stigmata of advanced liver disease, a low platelet count, elevated international normalized ratio (INR), or a fibrosis marker that corresponds to advanced fibrosis such as an APRI greater than 1.5. Up to 50% of people needing treatment will fulfill one of these criteria and can be started on antiviral medications without a liver biopsy. However, in others who have an elevated ALT level and an HBV DNA level of greater than 2000 IU/mL, but do not meet the previously mentioned criteria for advanced fibrosis, a liver biopsy might be necessary, as some of these patients will have mild or no fibrosis on biopsy, despite meeting ALT and HBV DNA criteria for active disease. This is important, because lifelong treatment with antiviral medication is often required. and the cost of oral antiviral agents for HBV is $5000 to $7000 per year. A percutaneous liver biopsy should be performed by an experienced clinician or radiologist, and it is imperative that the person doing the biopsy have a record of obtaining a sufficient amount of tissue so that an accurate interpretation by a pathologist can be made. This means a minimum of

2 cm of tissue using a 16-gauge needle that will hopefully yield at least 10 portal tracts. Below this sample size, the chance of sampling error will be greater than 10%. Liver biopsy is an invasive procedure, and, although the risk of serious complications is low, less than 1 per 1000 to 3000 biopsies, the procedure is wasted, and the patient has been inconvenienced if adequate tissue is not obtained. Furthermore, the wrong diagnostic interpretation due to inadequate tissue could lead to not prescribing antiviral medications to persons who warrant them and visa-versa.

Selection of Treatment Candidates and Criteria

Candidates for antiviral therapy, based on AASLD guidelines, include people with cirrhosis and those with evidence of moderate or severe inflammation or fibrosis as outlined previously.[23] Patients with decompensated cirrhosis should be treated only with a potent oral antiviral medication, as 30% to 50% of these patients may have a dramatic response and result in return of liver synthetic function accompanied by a return to fully compensated cirrhosis. In the rest, treatment may prolong survival long enough for a liver transplant to be performed in patients who meet criteria for transplantation. Treatment criteria for noncirrhotic patients are those in the immune-active phase of chronic HBV with an elevated ALT, HBV DNA greater than 2000 IU/mL (10,000 genomic copies/mL), and evidence of moderate or severe fibrosis or inflammation. In people who are HBeAg-positive, the goal of antiviral therapy is normalization of ALT, suppression of HBV DNA, loss of HBeAg, and seroconversion to anti-HBe. This occurs more frequently in persons with an ALT of at least twice the upper limit of normal. In patients who do not have this level of ALT elevation, less than 10% per year will experience HBeAg seroconversion. Patients who are HBeAg-positive and have normal ALT (immune-tolerant phase) will not benefit by treatment; HBeAg seroconversion will only infrequently occur. In those patients who are HBeAg-negative, the goal of treatment will be normalization of ALT and complete suppression of HBV DNA. HBeAg-negative persons in the inactive phase of HBV are not candidates for therapy.

Choice of Antiviral Medications for Chronic HBV

Seven antiviral medications are available for the treatment of chronic HBV (**Table 4**).[23] Three are considered first-line drugs: pegylated interferons, tenofovir, and entecavir.

Table 4
Medications available for the treatment of chronic hepatitis B infection

Medication	Administration	Effectiveness[a]	Risk of Resistance
First-Line			
Peg-interferon	Injectable	30%	None
Entecavir	Oral	>90% in naïve patients; less effective in lamivudine-experienced patients	<1% in naïve patients; 30% at 5 y in lamivudine-experienced patients
Tenofovir	Oral	>90%	<1%
Second-Line			
Lamivudine	Oral	<50%	70% at 5 y
Adefovir	Oral	<50%	30%–40%
Telbivudine	Oral	<70%	30% at 5 y
Emtricitabine	Oral	<50%	NA

[a] Suppression of DNA to undetectable, normalization of HBV DNA.

Pegylated interferon (peg-IFN) has the advantage of a limited treatment duration of 48 weeks, but the disadvantage of significant adverse effects and a success rate of only about 30% in people with HBeAg-positive and -negative immune active HBV. In those who do respond, however, subsequent loss of HBsAg occurs at a much higher rate than it does with oral antiviral medications. Recently, it has been found that the people who have the best chance of a response, about 50%, are those who are infected with HBV genotype A, and those with the worst chance of success are those infected with HBV genotype D (<10%).[38] This same study also found that the presence of the CC genotype for the interleukin (IL)-28 b gene, a commercially available test, also improves chance or response. Therefore, clinicians considering use of peg-IFN should consider doing at least HBV genotype testing and also IL-28 b testing. The oral antiviral medications for HBV all target the HBV reverse transcriptase enzyme. Tenofovir and entecavir should be the first-line drugs, as the other oral medications are either less potent and fail to suppress HBV DNA to undetectable levels or have a low barrier for developing resistance (see **Table 4**). Entecavir and tenofovir are equally effective, and have less than 1% risk of HBV resistance occurring over 5 to 6 years. Among patients who previously were treated with lamivudine, resistance to entecavir can develop in up to 20% after 5 years. Thus lamivudine-experienced persons should be treated with tenofovir, as resistance has not been a problem in this setting.

Length of Antiviral Treatment in Patients on Oral Antiviral Medications

In patients with HBeAg-positive HBV who are on oral antiviral therapy, treatment should continue until at least 6 to 12 months after the following have occurred: loss of HBeAg, appearance of anti-HBe, normalization of ALT, and undetectable levels of HBV DNA. In those who are anti-HBe positive at the onset of treatment, oral antiviral medications must be given indefinitely, because up to 90% of patients will relapse after stopping medication. A small percentage of persons on therapy will lose HBsAg, and if this occurs, antiviral medication may be stopped as long as HBV DNA is not detectable. In studies of patients with chronic HBV infection in whom spontaneous (without antiviral therapy) loss of HBsAg has occurred, cirrhosis did not develop in those who did not already have it, and the risk of HCC was significantly reduced but not eliminated.[13] It is assumed that the same good fortune will occur in persons who lose HBsAg while on antiviral therapy.

SPECIAL CONSIDERATIONS
HBV/HDV Coinfection

HDV is an incomplete viral agent that can only infect patients with chronic HBV.[39] HDV is an RNA virus that requires HBsAg as its envelope protein. Examples of this type of incomplete virus are found in plants, and HDV is the only one known in people. Patients with chronic HBV can develop HDV coinfection if they are exposed by a person who has both viruses. HDV coinfection can result in a severe acute type of hepatitis at time of initial exposure, with a fatality rate of approximately 15%. In those who recover from the acute hepatitis, a more rapid progression to cirrhosis is seen. HBV/HDV coinfection is most commonly found in the Mediterranean regions, parts of Russia, Greenland, and the Amazon basin. Unfortunately, oral antiviral medications have no effect, and peg-IFN is found to be effective in only about one-fourth of patients.[40] Long-term effects of peg-IFN may not be durable.[41] Even though HBV/HDV coinfection is uncommon, patients with chronic HBV should be screened for HDV by sending a test for antibody to HDV, especially if they were born in a region where HDV is common.

HBV/HIV Coinfection

From 5% to 15% of people infected with HIV are also infected with HBV.[42] Patients with this coinfection can experience more rapid progression of hepatic fibrosis as well as flares of hepatitis when the immune system is reconstituted on antiretroviral therapy (ART) if HBV is also not treated.[43] Recently, a higher incidence of acquired immunodeficiency syndrome (AIDS)-related complications and overall death rate was reported.[44,45] People taking ART that includes lamivudine as the only active drug against HBV have an up to a 90% chance of developing HBV resistance to lamivudine after 5 years, even if HIV RNA has remained nondetectable.[23,46] Practice guidelines and the World Health Organization (WHO) recommend that all people with HIV be screened for HBV and, if found to be coinfected, treated with a regimen that includes tenofovir and either lamivudine or emtricitabine.[23]

HBV/HCV Coinfection

In patients with HBV and HCV coinfection, the HCV virus usually predominates.[47] Multiple studies have shown that these patients have a much higher risk of developing HCC that appears to be either additive or synergistic.[48] If HCV is the dominant infection, either current treatment with interferon-based therapy or, with the advent of new potent direct-acting antiviral agents for HCV, treatment with one of these regimens to attempt to cure HCV first, and then manage HBV as outlined previously would be a rational strategy.

Reactivation of HBV with Cancer Chemotherapy or Immunosuppressive Therapy

HBsAg-positive patients who are undergoing chemotherapy for cancer or immunosuppressive therapy with potent agents such as tumor necrosis factor (TNF) inhibitors for rheumatic or autoimmune diseases are at great risk for reactivation of HBV regardless of which phase of the disease they are in.[49–51] Reactivation is characterized by the appearance or rise in the level of HBV DNA, which can be followed by a rise in ALT, liver cell injury, and even acute liver failure; reactivation can occur in up to 50% of these patients. HBV reactivation in patients who are HBsAg-negative but positive for anti-HBc is rare but can occur in those on potent chemotherapy for leukemia or lymphoma or who are receiving immunosuppressive medications that target lymphocytic B cells such as rituximab.[52] A systematic review of 550 HBsAg-positive patients who underwent chemotherapy for cancer found that over one-third had HBV reactivation; 13% of patients developed liver failure, and 5.5% of patients died.[53] The preemptive use of lamivudine in HBsAg-positive patients receiving chemotherapy in this analysis reduced the rate of reactivation by 79% to 100%, and no patient died of liver failure. The CDC and AASLD recommend screening patients for HBsAg, anti-HBs, and anti-HBc prior to undergoing chemotherapy or immunosuppressive therapy.[3,23] Those who are found to be HBsAg-positive should be started on an oral antiviral agent prior to starting treatment. The choice on antiviral agent has not been well studied, but in general, HBsAg-positive patients with low or absent HBV DNA can be treated with lamivudine or another second-line agent. Those with high levels of HBV DNA would likely benefit most from either entecavir or tenofovir. In those with absent or low levels of HBV DNA, prophylaxis should continue for 6 to 12 months after chemotherapy or inmmunotherapy is complete; in those with higher levels of HBV DNA, therapy should continue for a longer duration. In patients who are HBsAg-negative but anti-HBc-positive who are undergoing potent chemotherapy for leukemia or lymphoma or who are receiving drugs that target B cells such as rituximab, consideration for either use of prophylactic antiviral therapy at initiation of treatment or following HBV DNA levels and starting antiviral therapy if and when HBV DNA becomes positive should be considered. Precise screening and treatment regimens in these circumstances need to be worked out after carefully conducted studies have been performed.[54]

Management of HBV After Liver Transplantation

Only 2 decades ago, liver transplantation was contraindicated for HBV, because up to 50% of patients died of a severe form of hepatitis called fibrosing cholestasic hepatitis. However, the advent of intravenous hepatitis B immune globulin (HBIG) and oral antiviral agents has resulted in HBV being one of the conditions with the highest survival rates following liver transplant.[55] Several protocols for using antiviral therapy with and without HBIG are currently in use.

Screening for HCC

As mentioned earlier, patients with chronic HBV are at high risk for developing HCC, even if they do not have active liver disease. AASLD has developed practice guidelines that include recommendations for screening those at the highest risk of developing HCC (**Box 1**).[56] These recommendations are evidenced-based, for the most part; however, the recommendation to screen all men born in Africa above age 20 is not well supported; nor has cost effectiveness of this recommendation been worked out. In addition, several studies have shown that people who clear HBsAg after many years of positivity are still at a higher risk for HCC than the general population, although lower than those who remain HBsAg-positive.[13] Thus continuing screening in these individuals may be prudent, but the cost-effectiveness of doing so is unknown. The guidelines recommend screening those high-risk groups with liver ultrasound every 6 months. Some providers also include alpha-fetoprotein (AFP) testing, as AFP can rise rapidly in some patients months before lesions are detectable on ultrasound. AFP is fraught with a higher rate of false-positive and -negative results than ultrasound, however. AFP as a single tool for HCC screening in resource-constrained areas has also been shown to be more effective than no screening in detecting tumors early and in decreasing 5- and 10-year mortality.[28]

The Health Care Worker with Chronic HBV Infection

Recently, concern has been voiced regarding health care workers found to have chronic HBV infection, highlighted by cases of individuals having their acceptance to medical school revoked or being expelled from medical school when found to be HBsAg-positive. In March of 2013, the US Department of Justice ruled that a US medical school had violated the American with Disabilities Act by unlawfully excluding

---

Box 1
Persons with chronic HBV who are recommended by AASLD Practice Guidelines for regular surveillance with liver ultrasound every 6 months to detect HCC early at a treatable stage

- All men starting at age 40
- All women starting at age 50
- All people with family history of HCC
- All patients with cirrhosis
- People born in Africa starting at age 20[a]

   [a] Efficacy and cost-effectiveness data to support this recommendation are lacking.

applicants because they had hepatitis B. The CDC published in 2012 their updated recommendations for the management of HBV-infected health care workers and students.[57] These guidelines state that HBV infection alone should not disqualify persons from practice in any health field, nor should it be a reason for precluding them from applying to these professions. These guidelines address those infected health care workers performing exposure-prone procedures and recommended that an HBV level below 1000 IU/mL would be an appropriate level for health care facilities to allow an infected individual to perform exposure-prone procedures. For HBsAg-positive people above this level desiring to perform procedures, it would be reasonable to use antiviral therapy to reduce HBV DNA levels so that they could resume their specialties. However, no study to test this has been conducted.

SUMMARY

All providers, regardless of specialty, should perform screening for HBV on high-risk persons, especially those born in endemic countries. The primary care physician can perform the initial evaluation and follow-up of patients with chronic HBV by following the algorithm in this article and consulting with specialists when appropriate (see **Fig. 2**). Chronically infected patients should be followed on a regular basis, preferably every 6 months, with liver function tests, and when appropriate, HBV DNA levels. Those who meet the criteria for high risk for HCC should undergo liver ultrasound every 6 months. Powerful antiviral medications are available that can suppress but not cure HBV and result in resolution of liver inflammation and fibrosis, even cirrhosis, as well as decrease the risk of developing HCC. They should be used in those patients who meet the criteria outlined in the practice guidelines of the major liver societies.

REFERENCES

1. Lavanchy D. Hepatitis B virus epidemiology, disease burden, treatment, and current and emerging prevention and control measures. J Viral Hepat 2004; 11(2):97–107.
2. McMahon BJ. Epidemiology and natural history of hepatitis B. Semin Liver Dis 2005;25(Suppl 1):3–8.
3. Weinbaum CM, Mast EE, Ward JW. Recommendations for identification and public health management of persons with chronic hepatitis B virus infection. Hepatology 2009;49(5):S35–44.
4. McHugh JA, Cullison S, Apuzzio J, et al. Chronic hepatitis B infection: a workshop consensus statement and algorithm. J Fam Pract 2011;60(9):E1–8.
5. Beasley RP, Hwang LY, Lee GC, et al. Prevention of perinatally transmitted hepatitis B virus infections with hepatitis B virus infections with hepatitis B immune globulin and hepatitis B vaccine. Lancet 1983;2(8359):1099–102.
6. McMahon BJ, Alward WL, Hall DB, et al. Acute hepatitis B virus infection: relation of age to the clinical expression of disease and subsequent development of the carrier state. J Infect Dis 1985;151(4):599–603.
7. Bond WW, Favero MS, Petersen NJ, et al. Survival of hepatitis B virus after drying and storage for one week. Lancet 1981;1(8219):550–1.
8. McMahon BJ. Natural history of chronic hepatitis B. Clin Liver Dis 2009;14(3): 381–96.
9. Hoofnagle JH, Doo E, Liang TJ, et al. Management of hepatitis B: summary of a clinical research workshop. Hepatology 2007;45(4):1056–75.

10. McMahon BJ. The influence of hepatitis B virus genotype and subgenotype on the natural history of chronic hepatitis B. Hepatol Int 2009;3(2):334–42.
11. Ahn SH, Park YN, Park JY, et al. Long-term clinical and histological outcomes in patients with spontaneous hepatitis B surface antigen seroclearance. J Hepatol 2005;42(2):188–94.
12. Liaw YF, Sheen IS, Chen TJ, et al. Incidence, determinants and significance of delayed clearance of serum HBsAg in chronic hepatitis B virus infection: a prospective study. Hepatology 1991;13(4):627–31.
13. Simonetti J, Bulkow L, McMahon BJ, et al. Clearance of hepatitis B surface antigen and risk of hepatocellular carcinoma in a cohort chronically infected with hepatitis B virus. Hepatology 2010;51(5):1531–7.
14. Hadziyannis SJ, Vassilopoulos D. Hepatitis B e antigen-negative chronic hepatitis B. Hepatology 2001;34(4):617–24.
15. Beasley RP. Hepatitis B virus. The major etiology of hepatocellular carcinoma. Cancer 1988;61(10):1942–56.
16. McMahon BJ, Holck P, Bulkow L, et al. Serologic and clinical outcomes of 1536 Alaska natives chronically infected with hepatitis B virus. Ann Intern Med 2001;(135):759–68.
17. McMahon BJ. The natural history of chronic hepatitis B virus infection. Hepatology 2009;49(5):S45–55.
18. Livingston SE, Simonetti JP, McMahon BJ, et al. Hepatitis B virus genotypes in Alaska native people with hepatocellular carcinoma: preponderance of genotype F. J Infect Dis 2007;195(1):5–11.
19. Yang HI, Yeh SH, Chen PJ, et al. Associations between hepatitis B virus genotype and mutants and the risk of hepatocellular carcinoma. J Natl Cancer Inst 2008;100(16):1134–43.
20. Yang HI, Lu SN, Liaw YF, et al. Hepatitis B e antigen and the risk of hepatocellular carcinoma. N Engl J Med 2002;347(3):168–74.
21. Iloeje UH, Yang HI, Su J, et al. Predicting cirrhosis risk based on the level of circulating hepatitis B viral load. Gastroenterology 2006;130(3):678–86.
22. Goldstein ST, Zhou FJ, Hadler SC, et al. A mathematical model to estimate global hepatitis B disease burden and vaccination impact. Int J Epidemiol 2005;34(6):1329–39.
23. Lok AS, McMahon BJ. Chronic hepatitis B: update 2009. Hepatology 2009; 50(3):661–2.
24. European Association for the Study of the Liver. EASL clinical practice guidelines. Management of chronic hepatitis B European Association for the Study of the Liver. J Hepatol 2011;55:245–64.
25. Liaw YF, Leung N, Kao JH, et al. Asian-Pacific consensus statement on the management of chronic hepatitis B: a 2008 update. Hepatol Int 2008;2(3): 263–83.
26. Liaw YF, Sung JJ, Chow WC, et al. Lamivudine for patients with chronic hepatitis B and advanced liver disease. N Engl J Med 2004;351(15):1521–31.
27. Marcellin P, Gane E, Buti M, et al. Regression of cirrhosis during treatment with tenofovir disoproxil fumarate for chronic hepatitis B: a 5-year open-label follow-up study. Lancet 2013;381(9865):468–75.
28. McMahon BJ, Bulkow L, Harpster A, et al. Screening for hepatocellular carcinoma in Alaska natives infected with chronic hepatitis B: a 16-year population-based study. Hepatology 2000;32(4 Pt 1):842–6.
29. Castera L. Noninvasive Methods to Assess Liver Disease in Patients With Hepatitis B or C. Gastroenterology 2012;142(6):1293–302.e4.

30. Park SH, Kim CH, Kim DJ, et al. Usefulness of multiple biomarkers for the prediction of significant fibrosis in chronic hepatitis B. J Clin Gastroenterol 2011; 45(4):361–5.
31. Vallet-Pichard A, Mallet V, Nalpas B, et al. FIB-4: an inexpensive and accurate marker of fibrosis in HCV infection. Comparison with liver biopsy and fibrotest. Hepatology 2007;46(1):32–6.
32. Zhang YG, Wang BE, Wang TL, et al. Assessment of hepatic fibrosis by transient elastography in patients with chronic hepatitis B. Pathol Int 2010;60(4):284–90.
33. Castera L, Foucher J, Bernard PH, et al. Pitfalls of liver stiffness measurement: a 5-year prospective study of 13,369 examinations. Hepatology 2010;51(3): 828–35.
34. Fung J, Lai CL, Cheng C, et al. Mild-to-moderate elevation of alanine aminotransferase may increase liver stiffness measurement by transient elastography in patients with chronic hepatitis B. Hepatology 2009;50(4):971A.
35. McMahon BJ. Hepatitis B surface antigen (HBsAg): a 40-year-old hepatitis B virus seromarker gets new life. Gastroenterology 2010;139(2):380–2.
36. Brunetto MR, Olivari F, Colombatto P, et al. Use of HBsAg serum levels help to distinguish active from inactive HBV genotype D carriers. Gastroenterology 2010;139:483–90.
37. Chan HL, Wong VW, Wong GL, et al. A longitudinal study on the natural history of serum hepatitis B surface antigen changes in chronic hepatitis B. Hepatology 2010;52(4):1232–41.
38. Sonneveld MJ, Wong VW, Woltman AM. Polymorphisms near IL28B and serologic response to peginterferon in HBeAg-positive patients with chronic hepatitis B. Gastroenterology 2012;142(3):513–20.e1.
39. Hughes SA, Wedemeyer H, Harrison PM. Hepatitis delta virus. Lancet 2011; 378(9785):73–85.
40. Wedemeyer H, Yurdaydin C, Dalekos GN, et al. Peginterferon plus adefovir versus either drug alone for hepatitis delta. N Engl J Med 2011;364(4):322–31.
41. Triantos C, Kalafateli M, Nikolopoulou V, et al. Meta-analysis: antiviral treatment for hepatitis D. Aliment Pharmacol Ther 2012;35(6):663–73.
42. Kourtis AP, Bulterys M, Hu DJ, et al. HIV-HBV coinfection—a global challenge. N Engl J Med 2012;366(19):1749–52.
43. Thio CL, Seaberg EC, Skolasky R Jr, et al. HIV-1, hepatitis B virus, and risk of liver-related mortality in the multicenter cohort study (MACS). Lancet 2002; 360(9349):1921–6.
44. Chun HM, Roediger MP, Hullsiek KH, et al. Hepatitis B virus coinfection negatively impacts HIV outcomes in HIV seroconverters. J Infect Dis 2012;205(2): 185–93.
45. Nikolopoulos GK, Paraskevis D, Hatzitheodorou E, et al. Impact of Hepatitis B virus infection on the progression of AIDS and mortality in HIV-infected individuals: a cohort study and meta-analysis. Clin Infect Dis 2009;48(12):1763–71.
46. Benhamou Y, Bochet M, Thibault V, et al. Long-term incidence of hepatitis B virus resistance to lamivudine in human immunodeficiency virus-infected patients. Hepatology 2000;31(4):1030–1.
47. Liaw YF, Chen YC, Sheen IS, et al. Impact of acute hepatitis C virus superinfection in patients with chronic hepatitis B virus infection. Gastroenterology 2004; 126(4):1024–9.
48. Donato F, Boffetta P, Puoti M. A meta-analysis of epidemiological studies on the combined effect of hepatitis B and C virus infections in causing hepatocellular carcinoma. Int J Cancer 1998;75(3):347–54.

49. Hoofnagle JH. Reactivation of hepatitis B. Hepatology 2009;49(5):S156–65.
50. Yeo W, Chan PK, Zhong S, et al. Frequency of hepatitis B virus reactivation in cancer patients undergoing cytotoxic chemotherapy: a prospective study of 626 patients with identification of risk factors. J Med Virol 2000;62(3):299–307.
51. Carroll MB, Forgione MA. Use of tumor necrosis factor alpha inhibitors in hepatitis B surface antigen-positive patients: a literature review and potential mechanisms of action. Clin Rheumatol 2010;29(9):1021–9.
52. Leung C, Tsoi E, Burns G, et al. An argument for the universal prophylaxis of hepatitis B infection in patients receiving rituximab: a 7-year institutional experience of hepatitis screening. Oncologist 2011;16(5):579–84.
53. Loomba R, Rowley A, Wesley R, et al. Systematic review: the effect of preventive lamivudine on hepatitis B reactivation during chemotherapy. Ann Intern Med 2008;148(7):519–28.
54. Lok AS, Ward JW, Perrillo RP, et al. Reactivation of hepatitis B during immunosuppressive therapy: potentially fatal yet preventable. Ann Intern Med 2012; 156(10):743–5.
55. Buchanan C, Tran TT. Current status of liver transplantation for hepatitis B virus. Clin Liver Dis 2011;15(4):753–64.
56. Bruix J, Sherman M. Management of hepatocellular carcinoma: an update. Hepatology 2011;53(3):1020–2.
57. Holmberg SD, Suryaprasad A, Ward JW. Updated CDC recommendations for the management of hepatitis B virus-infected health-care providers and students. MMWR Recomm Rep 2012;61(3):1–12.

Review of Treatment Options for Nonalcoholic Fatty Liver Disease

Richele L. Corrado, MD[a], Dawn M. Torres, MD[b], Stephen A. Harrison, MD[c],*

KEYWORDS

- NAFLD • NASH • Epidemiology • Diagnosis • Treatment

KEY POINTS

- Nonalcoholic fatty liver disease (NAFLD) has become the most common cause of chronic liver disease in the United States and other western countries, and its prevalence has mirrored the rising obesity and diabetes mellitus epidemics.
- Among those with NAFLD, patients with nonalcoholic steatohepatitis (NASH) represent a large potential public health concern with risk for development of cirrhosis and hepatocellular carcinoma.
- NAFLD is characterized by hepatic steatosis as determined by imaging (ultrasound, MRI, or CT) or histology from liver biopsy.
- Patients are commonly first diagnosed by mild (1.5-fold to 4-fold) elevations in their serum aminotransferase, alanine aminotransferase, and aspartate aminotransferase, and/or by incidental radiographic evidence of steatosis.
- Although the future of NAFLD and NASH treatment has many promising agents, clinicians are currently faced with limited options and an emphasis on lifestyle modification.

INTRODUCTION

Nonalcoholic fatty liver disease (NAFLD), a major cause of chronic liver disease globally, encompasses a vast spectrum of disease that spans from isolated fatty liver (IFL) to nonalcoholic steatohepatitis (NASH), which is defined by necroinflammation with

Disclosures: Drs Corrado and Torres have nothing to disclose. Dr Harrison is a consultant for the Chronic Liver Disease Foundation and an Associate Editor for *Hepatology*.
Disclaimer: The views expressed herein are those of the authors and do not reflect the official policy or position of San Antonio Military Medical Center, the US Army Medical Department, the US Army Office of the Surgeon General, the Department of the Army, Department of Defense, or the US government.
[a] Department of Medicine, Walter Reed National Military Medical Center, 8901 Wisconsin Avenue, Bethesda, MD 20889-5600, USA; [b] Division of Gastroenterology, Department of Medicine, Walter Reed National Military Medical Center, 8901 Wisconsin Avenue, Bethesda, MD 20889-5600, USA; [c] Division of Gastroenterology, Department of Medicine, San Antonio Military Medical Center, 3551 Roger Brooke Drive, Fort Sam Houston, TX 78234, USA
* Corresponding author.
E-mail address: stephen.a.harrison.mil@mail.mil

hepatocyte injury and ballooning, along with a variable amount of fibrosis and potential for progression to cirrhosis. Over the past few decades, a rising NAFLD prevalence has reflected increasing obesity prevalence, suggesting a strong correlation between NAFLD and the escalating global obesity epidemic. Many experts now consider NAFLD to be a hepatic manifestation of metabolic syndrome, which is defined by the presence of three of the following: visceral obesity, elevated fasting plasma glucose, hypertension, hypertriglyceridemia, or low high-density lipoprotein levels.[1] This article details the pathogenesis of NAFLD, with an emphasis on the steps that result in the NASH phenotype, along with the current state of diagnosis and treatment of this common chronic liver disease.

EPIDEMIOLOGY

Global NAFLD prevalence rates ranges from 2.8% to 46%.[2,3] With time, NAFLD has become the most common cause of chronic liver disease in the United States and other western countries, and its prevalence has mirrored the rising obesity and diabetes mellitus (DM) epidemics. Recent global analysis estimates 1.5 million adults are overweight with a body mass index (BMI) of 25 kg/m^2 or greater, and 500 million adults are obese with a BMI of 30 kg/m^2 or greater.[4] In the United States, approximately 33.8% of the population is obese and 10.6% have DM type 2.[5]

The National Health and Nutrition Examination Surveys (NHANES) performed in the United States from 1988 to 2008 showed stable prevalence rates for chronic liver diseases, such as hepatitis B, hepatitis C, and alcoholic liver disease. However, the prevalence of NAFLD dramatically increased from 5.5% to 11%. Overall, NAFLD represented approximately 47% of all chronic liver disease in 1988, rising to 75% by 2008.[6] During this same time, the prevalence of several metabolic syndrome features, such as obesity, DM, insulin resistance (IR), and hypertension increased and, in one study, multivariate analysis found obesity to be an independent predictor of NAFLD.[7]

Estimating the true incidence and prevalence of NAFLD, specifically NASH, remains a challenge due both to the asymptomatic presentation of the disease as well as the lack of accurate and noninvasive diagnostic measurements. The prevalence of NAFLD was first estimated to be 36% in lean patients and 72% in obese patients in 1990 via autopsy. The prevalence of NASH in this same cohort was found to be 2.7% in lean patients and 18.5% in obese patients.[8] The evaluation of patients undergoing bariatric surgery confirmed the high prevalence rates among obese populations in which the prevalence of NAFLD and NASH was found to be 91% and 37%, respectively.[9] Of note, although NAFLD is strongly associated with obesity and other metabolic syndrome components, it can occur in patients without obesity and obesity does not guarantee the presence of NAFLD.

There have been several population based studies designed to ascertain NAFLD prevalence. In 2005, magnetic resonance spectroscopy (MRS) was used to identify asymptomatic steatosis in 31% of the 2100 adults in the Dallas Heart Study.[10] In 2011, a prospective study using ultrasound (US) evaluated 328 asymptomatic middle-aged subjects from Texas and found a 46% prevalence of NAFLD. Subsequent liver biopsies in patients with NAFLD demonstrated a 12.2% prevalence of NASH.[11] Studies have suggested that ethnicity plays a role in the development of NAFLD, with Hispanics at greatest risk, followed by whites, and then African Americans.[10–12] In adults, NAFLD is most commonly diagnosed during the fourth decade of life for men and sixth decade of life for women.[13] NAFLD is not only a disease of adults; it affects children and adolescents. Within these populations, NAFLD prevalence has proven to rise with increasing BMI.[14]

DEFINITION AND NATURAL HISTORY

NAFLD is characterized by hepatic steatosis as determined by imaging (US, MRI, or CT) or histology from liver biopsy. NAFLD includes IFL, indeterminate NASH, and NASH. Most patients with NAFLD have IFL or indeterminate NASH. IFL is defined by hepatic steatosis without evidence of hepatocyte injury or fibrosis, whereas indeterminate NASH is defined by nonspecific lobular or portal-based inflammation in the presence of hepatic steatosis but falls short of the histopathologic findings necessary to define NASH. Less common, yet more worrisome, is NASH, which is described as hepatic steatosis with histologic evidence of significant necroinflammation in the presence of hepatocyte injury (ballooning) with or without fibrosis.

Patients with NAFLD have a greater all-cause mortality compared with those without NAFLD,[15] with the most common causes of death being cardiovascular, malignancy, and liver-related disease, in order of decreasing frequency.[16,17] Advanced liver disease and the development of cirrhosis seems to be determined by histopathology because NASH has a higher risk of liver-related mortality than non-NASH,[7] and NASH with fibrosis has a worse prognosis than NASH without fibrosis. Characteristics related to increased fibrosis include DM, severe IR, BMI, weight gain greater than 5 kg, cigarette smoking, and rising alanine aminotransferase (ALT) and aspartate aminotransferase (AST) levels.[18,19] Finally, NASH patients with advanced fibrosis and cirrhosis are at the highest risk for the development of hepatocellular carcinoma (HCC). Age, obesity, and iron deposition are risk factors for developing HCC from NASH.[20]

ASSOCIATIONS AND PATHOGENESIS

As discussed previously, the link between NAFLD, obesity, DM and other metabolic syndrome components is widely accepted. Interestingly, recent studies support associations between hepatic steatosis and cardiovascular disease, obstructive sleep apnea, colonic adenomas, hyperuricemia, vitamin D deficiency (VDD), hyperferritinemia, hypothyroidism, pancreatic steatosis, and polycystic ovarian syndrome.[21–23] Recent research has focused on the myriad effects of vitamin D throughout the body beyond calcium homeostasis, including immune modulation, cell differentiation and proliferation, and the inflammatory response.[24] VDD has been implicated in several disease processes, including NAFLD in which low vitamin D levels have been independently associated with NAFLD and, in some instances, disease severity in NASH.[25] Vitamin D replacement represents an easy therapeutic target although study is required before it can be recommended as a treatment agent for NAFLD or NASH. However, if VDD is discovered, replacement is recommended typically as a dose of 50,000 IU weekly for 12 weeks with a subsequent low dose (400–800 IU) daily maintenance.

The pathogenesis of NAFLD was first described as the "two-hit hypothesis" by Day and James[26] in 1988. The first hit describes the development of hepatic steatosis from the dysregulation of fatty acid metabolism, which is largely affected by IR. A second insult was thought to drive the progression from bland steatosis to hepatocyte necroinflammation, ballooning, and fibrosis. Currently, however, the factors involved are poorly elucidated. As understanding of NAFLD evolved from the two-hit hypothesis, multiple pathways involving oxidative stress, inflammatory cytokine release, cellular autodigestion, and molecular endotoxins leading to apoptosis have shown to be important in the pathogenesis of NASH. In addition, the importance of genetic factors that promote hepatic steatosis, necroinflammation, or fibrinogenesis, as well as the human microbiome, has been strongly suggested by initial research. Further study is required to understand completely the complex and dynamic pathways leading to NASH cirrhosis.

CLINICAL MANIFESTATIONS AND DIAGNOSIS

Patients with NAFLD, including those with NASH, are most commonly asymptomatic on presentation, although some describe vague, nonspecific symptoms such as fatigue, nausea, and right upper quadrant pain. The presence of hepatomegaly is characteristic, although not always palpable, secondary to obesity. Patients are commonly first diagnosed by mild (1.5-fold to 4-fold) elevations in their serum amino-transferase, ALT, and AST, and/or by incidental radiographic evidence of steatosis. The accuracy of US, CT, and MRI for diagnosing NAFLD is high with greater than 90% sensitivity.[27] US is most commonly used for initial diagnosis because it is inexpensive, easily accessible, and safe. However, a higher threshold of steatosis, greater than 20%, is typically required for US to maintain a similar sensitivity and specificity to CT and MRI.[28] This suggests that US is inferior to CT or MRI for detecting lower amounts of steatosis.

Alkaline phosphatase and gamma-glutamyl transpeptidase elevations are often seen in patients with NAFLD with more advanced fibrosis; however, this is not diagnostic. In addition, data suggest that as disease severity increases, a concomitant rise in serum AST and in AST to ALT ratio can be seen.[29] Patients with NAFLD can demonstrate mild serum iron and ferritin elevations, as well as positive serum autoantibodies, such as antinuclear and anti–smooth muscle antibodies. Autoantibodies may be seen in approximately 20% of patients with NAFLD; however, their presence does not seem to correlate with presence or absence of NASH, or disease severity.[30] Although it is relatively easy to diagnosis NAFLD with history, clinical data, laboratory work, and/or radiologic imaging, distinguishing NASH from IFL remains a challenge because it requires liver biopsy for histopathology.

The ability to diagnosis NASH is crucial, especially concerning treatment options because these patients are at higher risk of fibrosis, progression to advanced liver disease, and cirrhosis. Although liver biopsy is the gold standard for diagnosing NASH, it is expensive and invasive. Consequently, advanced imaging techniques, specific laboratory tests, and predictive clinical scoring systems have been developed to help physicians. However, no single noninvasive test has proven equivalent or superior to liver biopsy. Scoring systems have been developed to predict the presence or absence of NASH, or the presence of advanced fibrosis. Myriad tests have been developed, including the NAFLD fibrosis score, European Liver Fibrosis score, the BARD score (BMI >28 kg/m², 1 point; AST or ALT $\geq$0.8, 2 points; and diabetes, 1 point), the FibroTest, and the NASHtest. Most are reliable for predicting minimal or advanced disease but fall short in most patients who have intermediate stage disease.

In the absence of a perfect noninvasive test that is easy to obtain and has high sensitivity and specificity, providers are often left to look for individual risk factors that may cumulatively point toward a diagnosis of NASH. Serum ferritin greater than 1.5 times the upper limit of normal has shown to predict more advanced NAFLD histology in both men and women.[31] Other clinical risk factors are outlined in **Fig. 1** and the authors recommend consideration of liver biopsy if at least two risk factors are present.

Once a liver tissue sample is obtained, NASH is usually defined by an experienced hepatopathologist as absent or present when there are minimal histologic criteria met, including macrovesicular steatosis, hepatocyte ballooning degeneration, and lobular inflammation.[32] Because present or absent is difficult to quantify in terms of disease

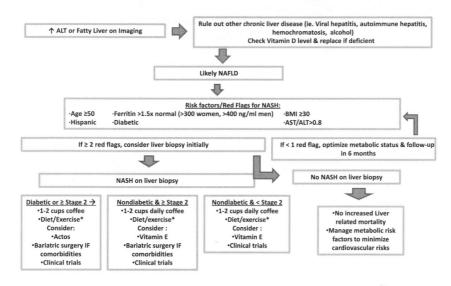

*See figure 2 for possible lifestyle modification approaches

Fig. 1. NAFLD diagnosis and treatment algorithm.

severity, the NAFLD activity score (NAS) was developed primarily as a research tool to monitor response to a medical intervention. With a scale of 0 to 9, levels greater than or equal to 5 are more often associated with NASH. However, this is by no means diagnostic and lower scores can be seen in patients who would meet NASH criteria. This was clearly outlined by Brunt and colleagues[33] who noted that, although there was a statistical correlation between NAS greater than or equal to 5 and an independent diagnosis of NASH by the pathologist, this was not the intent of the scoring system. NAS should only be used when looking at the response of a patient to an intervention, typically within the context of a research protocol.

TREATMENT

Because NAFLD has been considered the hepatic manifestation of the metabolic syndrome, most clinical efforts have focused on treating comorbidities such as obesity, IR, type II DM, and dyslipidemia. Lifestyle modifications, such as weight loss, diet, and exercise, have become the mainstay of treatment. The use of pharmacotherapeutic agents for NAFLD management is actively being examined with an emphasis placed on drugs that target IR, dyslipidemia, oxidative stress, proinflammatory cytokines, apoptosis, bacterial overgrowth, the angiotensin pathway, and other pathways thought important in the development of hepatic fibrosis.

Recently, studies have focused on treatments aimed at improving NASH rather than IFL because patients with NASH are at a greater risk for cirrhosis, HCC, and death.[34,35] Researchers continue to work toward a better understanding of the complicated pathogenesis of NASH and to focus drug development efforts. Various cohort studies and randomized controlled trials (RCTs) have attempted to establish ideal treatment and management plans; however, their conclusions are often limited by statistical power from small sample sizes and variable inclusion criteria.[36] Evidence of histologic improvement is ultimately needed to prove treatment success in those with NASH. Normalizing serum aminotransferase, improved glycemic control, and resolving radiographic steatosis do not always correlate with improvements in histology; therefore, treatment recommendations from studies that use such factors as primary endpoints cannot be made.

LIFESTYLE MODIFICATIONS

Lifestyle modifications encompass both diet and physical activity, and they have been the most promising treatment interventions identified for the first-line management of NAFLD.[35,37] Most studies evaluating the effects of diet and exercise on NAFLD, especially in subjects with NASH, have demonstrated that a weight loss of 3% to 7% was associated with decreased hepatic steatosis as proven by radiographic imaging or liver histology after lifestyle intervention.[38–41] Of these multiple studies recommending weight-loss interventions, many lack sufficient power due to low sample sizes and few provide biopsy-proven histologic changes.[38,39] The studies to date may be grouped into diet or exercise, or both.

Approaches using diet alone have included total calorie reduction as well as alteration of macronutrient composition. Kirk and colleagues,[42] randomized 22 obese subjects with greater than 50% steatosis per MRS to either a high-carbohydrate (>180 g/d) or low-carbohydrate (<50 g/d) caloric-restricted diet, then compared intrahepatic triglyceride (IHTG) content after 48 hours and again after approximately 7% weight loss, occurring after approximately 11 weeks. Despite comparable weight loss, IHTG content was significantly decreased in the low-carbohydrate group after 48 hours, yet similar in both groups after 7% weight loss. After 48 hours and study completion, subjects in the low-carbohydrate group had an increase in hepatic insulin sensitivity and a decrease in endogenous glucose production. Because IR is an important risk factor in the development of NAFLD, the improvements in insulin sensitivity seen in subjects receiving the low-carbohydrate diet may prove helpful in developing dietary interventions to prevent and treat hepatic steatosis.

Kistler and colleagues[43] retrospectively analyzed data from 1267 subjects enrolled in the NASH Clinical Research Network (CRN) and discovered that 54% of NAFLD subjects were sedentary, 20% met moderate physical activity standards, and 26% met vigorous activity recommendations. In subjects meeting vigorous activity standards, an average of 3 hours per week was spent mainly in treadmill running or aerobic step machines and, on average, they achieved 31.6 total metabolic equivalent for task (MET) hours per week. Interestingly, subjects in the vigorous activity group had significantly lower odds of having NASH and advanced fibrosis. Several other studies have supported this association between physical activity alone and improvements in hepatic steatosis with and without associated weight loss.[44–46] A systemic review and meta-analysis from 2011 reinforced that exercise independently reduces visceral adiposity,[47] which may be extended to improvements in hepatic steatosis. Debates between the types of physical activity (aerobic vs resistance) required to effect change in patients with NAFLD still exists. The 2011 meta-analysis did not reveal significant improvements after resistance therapy alone[47]; however, Hallsworth and colleagues[48] concluded that at least 8 weeks of resistance training, performed 45 to 60 minutes thrice weekly, was enough to moderately reduce intrahepatic lipid content. Larger RCTs are needed to establish the ideal exercise regimen required to induce histologic improvement of not just steatosis but also necroinflammation, hepatocyte ballooning, and fibrosis. In the interim, exercise of either aerobic or resistance training three to four times per week for 30 to 45 minutes of a moderate intensity seems a reasonable recommendation.

Diet and physical activity have also been investigated as a treatment pairing for NAFLD. Huang and colleagues[39] enrolled 23 subjects who had a BMI greater than 25 kg/m² and who were diagnosed NASH on biopsy in an intense dietary intervention program for 1 year with aims to reduce IR and weight. The dietary intervention recommended 1 to 2 pound weight loss per week and increased physical activity reaching at least 70% of the calculated target heart rate. Study subjects were required to maintain a food and exercise diary and attend nutritional counseling sessions with a registered dietitian. Primary endpoints of this study were a reduction in IR as assessed by the homeostatic model assessment (HOMA) score and histologic response as defined by a decrease in NAS by greater than or equal to 2 with at least one point from a non-steatosis component. Fifteen subjects completed the study and underwent follow-up liver biopsy; 60% had improved histology and IR. Subjects with histologic response also had an average of 7% weight loss compared with 2% weight loss in the histology nonresponders. Histologic responders also had greater physical activity as measured by the Paffenbarger Physical Activity Questionnaire. Although this was a successful study, it required intensive intervention with a high use of resources and was limited by the small overall number of subjects.

Intensive intervention seems necessary because treatment arms with more limited interventions using basic education about diet, exercise, and weight loss have not demonstrated sufficient weight loss to improve liver histology. Thirty-one obese subjects with evidence of NASH on biopsy were assigned to structured basic education versus an intense lifestyle change program. This program encouraged at least 200 minutes per week of moderate-intensity physical activity for 48 weeks in addition to providing specific, calorie-directed dietary guidance and behavioral support to maintain program inherence. Thirty participants completed the 48-week study. The control arm had a 0.2% weight loss compared with 9.3% in the intensive arm, and the intensive arm exhibited greater reductions in NAS. Overall, a weight loss of 7% or greater was correlated with improved histologic steatosis, necrosis, and inflammation, although not fibrosis.[36]

Although dietary changes that result in weight loss seem to improve steatosis and necroinflammation, no specific dietary macronutrient recommendations or combination diet and exercise therapy have been made in the recent tri-society (American Association for the Study of Liver Diseases, American College of Gastroenterology, and the American Gastroenterological Association) practice guideline.[35] A recent RCT performed by Eckard and colleagues[49] assessed four lifestyle modifications: (1) standard of care to include diet education, (2) low-fat diet (20% fat, 60% carbohydrate, 20% protein) with moderate exercise, (3) moderate-fat or low processed-carbohydrate diet (30% fat, 50% carbohydrate, 20% protein) with moderate exercise, and (4) moderate exercise only. Fifty-six participants with biopsy-proven NAFLD were enrolled and 41 completed the 6-month study with repeat liver biopsies to assess histologic change after intervention. All subgroups demonstrated a significant decrease in NAS although there was no significantly superior group. No subgroup attained a weight loss of 5% or greater and subjects in the moderate exercise group experienced mild weight gain. Differences between the low-fat and moderate-fat diets were not identified, but review of food logs proved that roughly 50% of participants did not comply with their recommended dietary parameters. This trial again supported the efficacy of lifestyle intervention but emphasized the difficulty with subject compliance even with the frequent follow-up of a clinical trial. Most of the study participants did not lose a significant amount of weight yet NAS still improved throughout subgroups. These findings have led some investigators to suggest that healthier lifestyles, even in the absence of weight loss, may be beneficial for patients with NAFLD.[50]

Data taken from the NASH CRN analyzed the effects of fructose on NAFLD severity in 427 subjects and concluded that daily fructose consumption was associated with increased fibrosis.[51,52] Analysis of dietary macronutrient components has also suggested that high amounts (>10% of total energy) of saturated fat, particularly trans-saturated fats, contributes to IR and potential to increased NASH risk.[53,54] Although further study is necessary to clarify the role of both fructose and saturated fat in NAFLD, the degree of evidence available at this point is strong enough to recommend limiting intake of both in NAFLD populations.

Certain food and nutrients have also been investigated for their potentially beneficial effects in NAFLD. In particular, omega-3 fatty acids and coffee have shown some promise in early study. In the rodent model, omega-3 fatty acid supplementation improved insulin sensitivity and decreased IHTG content as well as steatohepatitis.[55] These findings prompted several RCTs in humans that evaluated omega-3 supplementation in NAFLD subjects. Overall results demonstrated decreased ALT, triglycerides, HOMA levels, and steatosis per radiographic imaging, as well as decreased tumor necrosis factor α (TNF-α) levels, although the studies are lacking in defined histopathologic endpoints.[56–58] Although omega-3 fatty acids have shown initial promise for patients with NAFLD, the tri-society guideline considers their use for the treatment of NAFLD premature and proposes more RCTs with adequate sample sizes and specified histopathologic endpoints. The risks, if any, of long-term omega-3 supplementation have not been defined and it does seem reasonably safe.[59] The authors would not discourage supplementation if a patient independently chose to do so but the data are insufficient to warrant prescription of omega-3 to patients with NAFLD.

Caffeinated coffee is comprised of several bioactive compounds with favorable effects on health.[60] Studies have linked its consumption with decreased hepatic fibrosis in patients with chronic liver disease, especially hepatitis C[61] and HCC.[62] A recent cross-sectional study found an inverse relationship between the amount of caffeinated coffee consumed and hepatic fibrosis in NASH patients.[63] It is unclear which of the greater than 1000 substances in coffee provide the most benefit and it does not necessarily seem correlated to the amount of caffeine because a study comparing regular coffee drinkers with those who consumed espresso showed less fibrosis in the regular coffee drinkers.[64] At this point, moderate daily unsweetened coffee may be considered a reasonable adjunct to a multidisciplinary treatment plan for patients with NAFLD with the understanding that a controlled prospective study is required to determine if coffee can truly be a therapy for patients with NAFLD.[65]

BARIATRIC SURGERY

The use of bariatric surgery in patients with NAFLD has become an interesting treatment consideration because it induces considerable weight loss. Mathurin and colleagues[66] conducted a 5-year prospective study to evaluate NASH and fibrosis in 381 subjects who underwent bariatric surgery. Postsurgery, laboratory data, and liver biopsies showed decreased steatosis and hepatocyte ballooning in conjunction with improved insulin sensitivity, although fibrosis seemed to worsen. Numerous studies have followed with most showing some degree of histologic improvement, including fibrosis as shown most recently in a cohort of 78 morbidly obese subjects who underwent gastric bypass.[67] However, the studies were heterogenous with varying inclusion criteria and endpoints. In 2010, a Cochrane review[68] determined that the evidence for bariatric surgery in the management of NAFLD was limited and inconclusive due to the lack of well-structured trials with sufficient sample sizes and, in agreement, the tri-society guideline states that is premature to use bariatric surgery as a treatment option for NASH.[35] Bariatric surgery may be a reasonable option in individuals with comorbid conditions in addition to NASH that would justify the risk and cost of the procedure.

PHARMACOLOGIC AGENTS

Pharmacotherapy is an appealing treatment of NAFLD and, specifically, NASH because there is a general acceptance of the need for chronic medications associated with many other facets of the metabolic syndrome, such as hypertension or hyperlipidemia. Unfortunately, there is no medical therapy approved by the Food and Drug Administration (FDA) for NASH, although many have been investigated and some have shown promise in early study. These medications may be grouped by mechanism of action; some promote general weight loss and others are directed at pathways related to the pathogenesis of NASH, as well as fibrinogenesis.

Weight Loss Medications

Pharmacologic agents that induce weight loss have been investigated as potential treatment options for NAFLD. Orlistat, an enteric lipase inhibitor, showed potential in pilot studies and prompted two RCTs for further evaluation. Zelber-Sagi and colleagues[69] found that orlistat decreased serum ALT levels and US evidence of hepatic steatosis, but weight loss and histologic changes between the groups were not statistically significant. Harrison and colleagues[70] found no difference in the amount of weight lost by subjects taking orlistat or placebo but did associate a greater than or equal to 9% weight loss with reduced steatosis and inflammation. Both studies failed to demonstrate improvement in liver fibrosis. Motivation for continued trials ceased in 2009 after the FDA released a postmarketing warning about rare reports of severe liver injury as well as issues with patient tolerance secondary to the oily diarrhea associated with fatty meals.

Sibutramine, a serotonin and norepinephrine reuptake inhibitor, induces weight loss by decreasing appetite and increasing satiety.[71] The studies exploring its use in subjects with NAFLD are limited, but one study did report that it reduced aminotransferase and improved steatosis on US.[72] However, safety concerns about the use sibutramine exist after reported increased blood pressure in subjects while concurrently inducing weight loss.[73] In addition, there were increased cardiovascular events in a larger trial that resulted in its removal from the European and American markets.[74] The centrally and peripherally acting cannabinoid type 1 receptor antagonist, rimonabant, was met with a similar fate after it was associated with increased rates of suicide.[75] Future study is required with the two most recently approved weight loss medications: lorcaserin (Lorqess, Belviq), a selective serotonin 2c receptor agonist, and the combination formulation of phentermine and topiramate (Qnexa).

Insulin Sensitizing Agents

Many studies have investigated the use of diabetic medications including metformin, thiazolidinediones (TZDs), and incretin mimetics as potential treatment options for patients with NAFLD. The studies with metformin have generally been disappointing despite its beneficial effects on glucose homeostasis and modest weight loss. A recent meta-analysis concluded that the drug did not improve serum aminotransferase or liver histology in comparison to lifestyle modifications alone,[76] and the tri-society guideline reinforces those findings by not recommending its use in treatment specifically for NASH.[35]

TZDs, which are peroxisomal proliferator-activated receptor (PPAR)-γ agonists, decrease hepatic lipogenesis, increase insulin sensitivity, and stimulate hepatic fatty aid oxidation. A 2010 review, which looked at three uncontrolled trials[77–79] and five RCTs,[80] examined the usefulness of TZDs (rosiglitazone and pioglitazone) for the treatment of NASH. This analysis concluded that glitazones reduce hepatic steatosis, necroinflammation, and hepatocyte ballooning; however, they do not consistently improve liver fibrosis.[81–85] Although arguably one of the most efficacious therapies that are currently available, their side effects have limited their widespread acceptance and use. Despite ability to decrease steatohepatitis, TZDs have been associated with weight gain, decreased bone density, increased fractures, higher rates of heart failure, and possibly bladder cancer.[79] Rosiglitazone lost popularity in 2007 after the FDA released a black box warning connecting it with high rates of myocardial ischemia and infarct. The tri-society guideline states that pioglitazone can be used in biopsy-proven NASH, although they caution its use because long-term safety and efficacy outcomes are indeterminate.[33] In addition to the TZDs, there has been preliminary study using agents that are combination PPAR agonists. PPAR-δ agonists have been shown to improve dyslipidemia and increase fat oxidation in muscle and PPAR-α agonists increase fatty acid oxidation in multiple tissue types.[86] Although in early trials, dual PPARα/δ agonists improved IR and dyslipidemia. Further study with this and other combination PPAR agonists are ongoing although some enthusiasm for these agents have been dampened by potential renal and cardiovascular side effects seen in some early clinical trials.

Incretin mimetics (exenatide and liraglutide) are the most recent diabetic medications that seem promising for the treatment of NASH. These glucagon-like peptide-1 receptor (GLP-1R) agonists are cardioprotective agents that decrease IR, weight gain, and inflammation. Animal studies with exenatide have exhibited improved insulin sensitivity and hepatic steatosis in addition to decreasing fat accumulation in the liver by inhibition of hepatic lipogenesis.[87] Exenatide use in several human case studies has demonstrated decreased aminotransferase and hepatic steatosis[88] with some histologic improvement, although this was not statistically significant possibly due to small sample size.[89] Although encouraging, RCTs are still needed to investigate further the effects of these agents on NAFLD.

Lipid-Lowering Agents

Lipid-lowering agents, such as statins, fenofibrates, and ezetimibe, are commonly used to treat dyslipidemia, especially in patients with cardiovascular risk factors. Patients with dyslipidemia often suffer from obesity, diabetes, and other components of metabolic syndrome, including NAFLD. In the past, these agents, particularly statins, were avoided in patients with liver disease for fear of causing aminotransferase elevations and perpetuating liver injury. A review by Nseir and colleagues[90] analyzed case studies for the past 32 years and concluded that statins, fibrates, and ezetimibe are all safe to use in patients with NAFLD, and they may actually improve hepatic steatosis. Studies in NASH populations have been limited to pilot trials in which only modest histologic improvement has been demonstrated.[91,92] The tri-society guideline supports the use of statins in patients with NAFLD only for the treatment of dyslipidemia. More evidence-based research is needed before they should be used specifically for NASH; however, they are recommended as primary treatment of dyslipidemia in all patients with NAFLD.[35]

Antioxidants

The effects of oxidative stress and its associated proinflammatory cytokines are considered potential contributors to steatohepatitis. This hypothesis has prompted investigation into the use of antioxidant agents for the treatment of NAFLD. Vitamin E is the most commonly studied agent with generally beneficial results in adult NASH. A small RCT with 49 subjects found significant improvements in liver fibrosis but not inflammation in subjects treated with Vitamin E 1000 IU and vitamin C 1000 mg daily.[93] A subsequent larger trial in nondiabetic NASH subjects randomly assigned 247 subjects to either 30 mg pioglitazone daily, 800 IU vitamin E daily, or placebo. This trial demonstrated that vitamin E lead to significant improvements in hepatic steatosis and lobular inflammation but no change in fibrosis.[85] Although once considered a completely benign therapy, vitamin E has recently been reported to increase cardiovascular risk, all-cause mortality,[94] and prostate cancer rates.[95] Despite these negative associations, the tri-society guideline suggests the use of vitamin E in nondiabetics should be considered first-line therapy for NASH, although they caution its use in diabetics without biopsy-proven NASH.[35]

Other antioxidants, such as betaine and N-acetyl-cysteine (NAC), have also been investigated in small trials. Betaine is a choline metabolite that increases s-adenosyl methionine (SAM) levels and decreases oxidative stress. Elevated SAM levels in animal studies suggest steatohepatitis improvement.[96] However, a 1-year RCT assessing the effects of 20 g daily betaine versus placebo did not demonstrate promising rates. Abdelmalek and colleagues[97] noted an improvement in steatosis in betaine-treated subjects compared with placebo but no change in NAS score or fibrosis stage. Rat studies have linked the use of NAC to improvements in liver fibrosis,[98] yet two small human studies showed only aminotransferase improvements with NAC; neither study performed posttreatment biopsy.[99,100] Betaine and NAC cannot be recommended at this time.

Cytoprotective Agents

Cytoprotective agents are presumed to decrease proinflammatory cytokines and prevent cellular apoptosis. Multiple studies evaluating ursodeoxycholic acid (UDCA) effects on NALFD subjects have yielded conflicting results.[101–103] In lieu of convincing study data and recent reports of UDCA causing increased mortality in primary sclerosing cholangitis patients, the tri-society practice guideline does not recommend UDCA for NAFLD treatment.[35]

Pentoxifylline (PTX) is a xanthine derivative shown to decrease inflammation by inhibiting TNF-α. Human pilot studies have documented some reductions in steatosis, inflammation, ballooning,[104,105] and fibrosis[106] with PTX, although further RCTs are needed to assess the use of PTX as a potential agent for NAFLD treatment.

New Therapeutics of Interest

The intestinal microbiome refers to an individual's gut flora and recent evidence has suggested this to be significant in several chronic diseases, including NAFLD. Oxidative stress from the overgrowth of gastrointestinal bacteria has recently been proposed as a contributor to the development of NAFLD. Probiotics administered to mice have improved liver histology and reduced aminotransferases.[107] Similarly, small pilot studies in humans have shown decreased aminotransferase and decreased markers of oxidative stress.[108] In the absence of histologic data, the use of probiotics in the management of NAFLD cannot yet be recommended and future study is required.

The renin-angiotensin system (RAS) is most commonly known for its regulation of blood pressure and fluid balance, but it also can increase IR and adipose tissue proliferation. RAS blockade with angiotensin II receptor blockers (ARBs) improves hypertension, heart failure, and chronic kidney disease. ARBs in obese rodent studies have

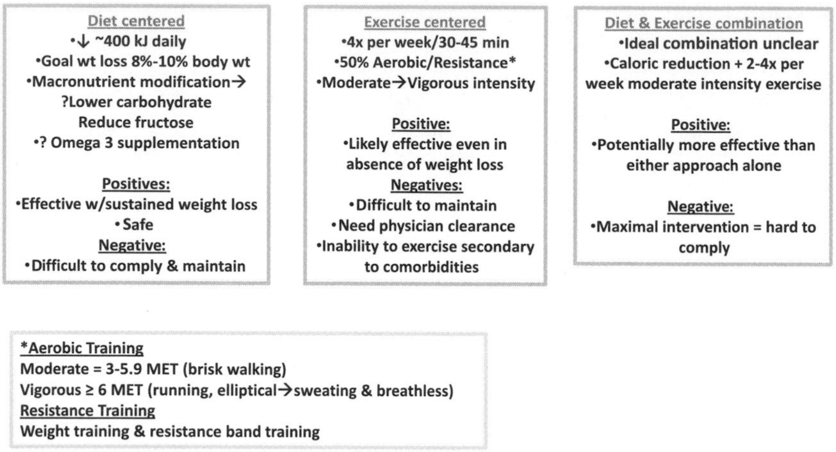

Diet centered	Exercise centered	Diet & Exercise combination
•↓ ~400 kJ daily •Goal wt loss 8%-10% body wt •Macronutrient modification→ ?Lower carbohydrate Reduce fructose •? Omega 3 supplementation **Positives:** •Effective w/sustained weight loss • Safe **Negative:** •Difficult to comply & maintain	•4x per week/30-45 min •50% Aerobic/Resistance* •Moderate→Vigorous intensity **Positive:** •Likely effective even in absence of weight loss **Negatives:** •Difficult to maintain •Need physician clearance •Inability to exercise secondary to comorbidities	•Ideal combination unclear •Caloric reduction + 2-4x per week moderate intensity exercise **Positive:** •Potentially more effective than either approach alone **Negative:** •Maximal intervention = hard to comply

*Aerobic Training
Moderate = 3-5.9 MET (brisk walking)
Vigorous ≥ 6 MET (running, elliptical→sweating & breathless)
Resistance Training
Weight training & resistance band training

Fig. 2. NAFLD lifestyle modification approaches. MET, metabolic equivalent for task; wt, weight.

demonstrated less hepatic stellate cell activation,[109] which can contribute to fibrosis formation. The impacts of ARBs in humans support reduced IR. However, liver histologic benefits have yet to be established and the one large study to date using losartan in combination with rosiglitazone failed to show a benefit compared with rosiglitazone alone.[110] More trials evaluating ARB effects on steatohepatitis and fibrosis are essential before these drugs can be recommended specifically for the treatment of NAFLD.

Bile acid metabolism is a newer area of NAFLD research. The secretion of bile acids occurs in response to food intake and they play an important role in both lipid and glucose metabolism via binding with nuclear hormone receptors such as the farnesoid X receptor (FXR). FXR agonists improve insulin sensitivity and suppress proinflammatory genes in a manner potentially beneficial for patients with NASH.[111] Obeticholic acid is an FXR agonist that recently improved insulin sensitivity, as well as markers of liver inflammation and fibrosis, compared with placebo in a cohort of NAFLD subjects.[112] The future results of the FXR Ligand NASH Treatment (FLINT) study, a phase IIb RCT that includes liver histologic endpoints, are eagerly anticipated.

SUMMARY

Although the future of NAFLD and NASH treatment has many promising agents, clinicians are currently faced with limited options with an emphasis on lifestyle modification. **Figs. 1** and **2** summarize current practices for the diagnosis and treatment of NAFLD with the understanding that each patient's treatment must be customized to their comorbidities, exercise tolerance, and willingness to comply with therapy.

REFERENCES

1. Alberti KG, Eckel RH, Grundy SM, et al. Harmonizing the metabolic syndrome: a joint interim statement of the International Diabetes Federation Task Force on Epidemiology and Prevention; National Heart, Lung, and Blood Institute; American Heart Association; World Heart Federation; International Atherosclerosis Society; and International Association for the Study of Obesity. Circulation 2009;120:1640–5.

2. Lazo M, Clark JM. The epidemiology of nonalcoholic fatty liver disease: a global perspective. Semin Liver Dis 2008;28:339–50.
3. Lazo M, Hernandez R, Eberhardt MS, et al. Prevalence of nonalcoholic fatty liver disease in the United States: the Third National Health and Nutritional Examination Survey, 1988-1994. Am J Epidemiol 2013;178:38–45.
4. Finucane MM, Stevens GA, Cowan MJ, et al. National, regional, and global trends in body-mass index since 1980: systematic analysis of health examination surveys and epidemiological studies with 960 country-years and 9.1 million participants. Lancet 2011;377(9765):557–67.
5. Flegal KM, Carroll MD, Ogden CL, et al. Prevalence and trends in obesity among US adults, 1999–2008. JAMA 2010;303:235–41.
6. Younossi ZM, Stepanova M, Afendy M, et al. Changes in the prevalence of the most common causes of chronic liver diseases in the United States from 1988 to 2008. Clin Gastroenterol Hepatol 2011;9(6):524–30.
7. Stepanova M, Rafiq N, Makhlouf H, et al. Predictors of all-cause mortality and liver-related morality in patients with non-alcoholic fatty liver disease. Dig Dis Sci 2013;58:3017–23.
8. Wanless IR, Lentz JS. Fatty liver hepatitis (steatohepatitis) and obesity: an autopsy study with analysis of risk factors. Hepatology 1990;12:1106–10.
9. Machado M, Marques-Vidal P, Cortez-Pinto H. Hepatic histology in obese patients undergoing bariatric surgery. J Hepatol 2006;45:600–6.
10. Szczepaniak L, Nurenburg P, Leonard D, et al. Magnetic resonance spectroscopy to measure hepatic triglyceride content: prevalence of hepatic steatosis in the general population. Am J Physiol Endocrinol Metab 2005;288:462–8.
11 Williams CD, Stengel J, Asike MI, et al. Prevalence of nonalcoholic fatty liver disease and nonalcoholic steatohepatitis among a largely middle-aged population utilizing ultrasound and liver biopsy: a prospective study. Gastroenterology 2011;140:124–31.
12. Browning JD, Szczepaniak LS, Dobbins R, et al. Prevalence of hepatic steatosis in an urban population in the United States: impact of ethnicity. Hepatology 2004;40:1387–95.
13. Ruhl CE, Everhart JE. Epidemiology of nonalcoholic fatty liver disease. Clin Liver Dis 2004;8:501–19.
14. Ogden CL, Carroll MD, Curtin LR, et al. Prevalence of high body mass index in children and adolescents, 2007–2008. JAMA 2010;303:242–9.
15. Ruhl CE, Everhart JE. Elevated serum alanine aminotransferase and gamma-glutamyltransferase and mortality in the United States population. Gastroenterology 2009;136:477–85.
16. Dam-Larson S, Becker U, Franzmann MG, et al. Final results of a long-term, clinical follow up in fatty liver patients. Scand J Gastroenterol 2009;44:1236–43.
17. Soderberg C, Stal P, Askling J, et al. Decreased survival of subjects with elevated liver function tests during a 28-year follow-up period. Hepatology 2010;51:595–602.
18. Adams LA, Sanderson S, Lindor KD, et al. The histological course of nonalcoholic fatty liver disease: a longitudinal study of 103 patients with sequential liver biopsies. Hepatology 2005;42:132–8.
19. Zein CO, Unalp A, Colvin R, et al. Smoking and severity of hepatic fibrosis in nonalcoholic fatty liver disease. J Hepatol 2011;54:753–9.
20. Starley BQ, Calcagno CJ, Harrison SA. Nonalcoholic fatty liver disease and hepatocellular carcinoma: weighty connection. Hepatology 2012;51:1820–32.

21. Liangpunsakul S, Chalasani N. Is hypothyroidism a risk factor for non-alcoholic steatohepatitis? J Clin Gastroenterol 2003;37:340–3.
22. Baranova A, Tran TP, Birerdnc A, et al. Systemic review: association of polycystic ovary syndrome with metabolic syndrome and non-alcoholic fatty liver disease. Aliment Pharmacol Ther 2011;33:801–14.
23. Lee YI, Lim YS, Park HS. Colorectal neoplasms in relation to non-alcoholic fatty liver disease in Korean women: a retrospective cohort study. J Gastroenterol Hepatol 2012;27:91–5.
24. Kwok RM, Torres DM, Harrison SA. Vitamin D and NAFLD: is it more than just an association? Hepatology 2013;58:1166–74.
25. Targher G, Bertolini L, Scala L. Associations between serum 25-hydroxyvitamin D3 concentrations and liver histology in patients with nonalcoholic fatty liver disease. Nutr Metab Cardiovasc Dis 2007;17:517–24.
26. Day CP, James OF. Steatohepatitis: a tale of two "hits"? Gastroenterology 1998; 114:842–5.
27. Schwenzer NF, Springer F, Schrami C, et al. Non-invasive assessment and quantification of liver steatosis by ultrasound, computed tomography and magnetic resonance. J Hepatol 2009;51:433–45.
28. Hernaez R, Lazo M, Bonekamp S, et al. Diagnosis accuracy and reliability of ultrasonography for the detection of fatty liver: a meta-analysis. Hepatology 2011;54:1082–90.
29. Palekar NA, Naus R, Larson SP, et al. Clinical model for distinguishing nonalcoholic steatohepatitis from simple steatosis in patients with nonalcoholic fatty liver disease. Liver Int 2006;26(2):151–6.
30. Vuppalanchi R, Gould RJ, Wilson LA, et al. Clinical significance of serum autoantibodies in patients with NAFLD: results from the nonalcoholic steatohepatitis clinical research network. Hepatol Int 2011. [Epub ahead of print].
31. Kowdley KV, Belt P, Wilson LA, et al. Serum ferritin is an independent predictor of histologic severity and advanced fibrosis in patients with nonalcoholic fatty liver disease. Hepatology 2012;55(1):77–85.
32. Brunt EM. Nonalcoholic steatohepatitis: definition and pathology. Semin Liver Dis 2001;21:3–16.
33. Brunt EM, Kleiner DE, Behling C, et al. Misuse of scoring systems. Hepatology 2011;54:369–70.
34. Lam B, Younossi ZM. Treatment options for nonalcoholic fatty liver disease. Therap Adv Gastroenterol 2010;3:121–37.
35. Chalasani N, Younossi Z, Lavine JE, et al. The diagnosis and management of non-alcoholic fatty liver disease: practice guideline by the American Association for the Study of Liver Diseases, American College of Gastroenterology, and the American Gastroenterological Association. Hepatology 2012;55:2005–23.
36. Torres DM, Williams CD, Harrison SA. Features, diagnosis, and treatment of nonalcoholic fatty liver disease. Clin Gastroenterol Hepatol 2012;10:837–58.
37. Harrison S, Day C. Benefits of lifestyle modification in NAFLD. Gut 2007;56: 1760–9.
38. Promrat K, Kleiner D, Niemeier H, et al. Randomized controlled trial testing the effects of weight loss on nonalcoholic steatohepatitis. Hepatology 2010;51:121–9.
39. Huang MA, Greenson JK, Chao C, et al. One-year intense nutritional counseling results in histological improvement in patients with non-alcoholic steatohepatitis: a pilot study. Am J Gastroenterol 2005;100:1072–81.
40. Cowin GJ, Jonsson JR, Bauer JD, et al. Magnetic resonance imaging and spectroscopy for monitoring liver steatosis. J Magn Reson Imaging 2008;28:937–45.

41. Lazo M, Solga SF, Horska A, et al. Effect of a 12-month intensive lifestyle intervention on hepatic steatosis in adults with type 2 diabetes. Diabetes Care 2010; 33:2156–63.
42. Kirk E, Reeds DN, Finck BN, et al. Dietary fat and carbohydrates differentially alter insulin sensitivity during caloric restriction. Gastroenterology 2009;136: 1552–60.
43. Kistler KD, Brunt EM, Clark JM, et al. Physical activity recommendations, exercise intensity, and histological severity of nonalcoholic fatty liver disease. Am J Gastroenterol 2011;106:460–8.
44. St George A, Bauman A, Johnston A, et al. Independent effects of physical activity in patients with nonalcoholic fatty liver disease. Hepatology 2009;50: 68–76.
45. Perseghin G, Lattuada G, Cobelli De, et al. Habitual physical activity is associated with intrahepatic fat content in humans. Diabetes Care 2007;30:683–8.
46. Johnson NA, Sachinwalla T, Walton DW, et al. Aerobic exercise training reduces hepatic and visceral lipids in obese individuals without weight loss. Hepatology 2009;50:1105–12.
47. Ismail I, Keating SE, Baker MK, et al. A systemic review and meta-analysis of the effect of aerobic vs resistance exercise training on visceral fat. Obes Rev 2012; 13:68–91.
48. Hallsworth K, Fattakhova G, Hollingsworth KG, et al. Resistance exercise reduces liver fat and its mediators in nonalcoholic fatty liver disease independent of weight loss. Gut 2011;60:1278–83.
49. Eckard C, Cole R, Lockwood J, et al. Prospective histopathologic evaluation of lifestyle modification in nonalcoholic fatty liver disease: a randomized trial. Ther Advances Gastroenterol 2013;6(4):249–59.
50. Wang RT, Koretz RL, Yee HF Jr. Is weight reduction an effective therapy for nonalcoholic fatty liver? A systematic review. Am J Med 2003;115:554–9.
51. Abdelmalek MF, Suzuki A, Guy C, et al. Increased fructose consumption is associated with fibrosis severity in patients with nonalcoholic fatty liver disease. Hepatology 2010;51:1961–71.
52. Ouyang X, Cirillo P, Sautin Y, et al. Fructose consumption as a risk factor for nonalcoholic fatty liver disease. J Hepatol 2008;48:993–9.
53. Musso G, Gambino R, De Michieli F, et al. Dietary habits and their relations to insulin resistance and postprandial lipemia in nonalcoholic steatohepatitis. Hepatology 2003;37:909–16.
54. Zivkovic AM, German JB, Sanyal AJ. Comparative review of diets for the metabolic syndrome: implications for non-alcoholic fatty liver disease. Am J Clin Nutr 2007;86:285–300.
55. Svegliati-Baroni G, Candelaresi C, Saccomanno S, et al. A model of insulin resistance and nonalcoholic steatohepatitis in rats: role of peroxisome proliferator-activated receptor-alpha and n-3 polyunsaturated fatty acid treatment on liver injury. Am J Pathol 2006;169:846–60.
56. Tilg H, Moschen AR. Adipocytokines: mediators linking adipose tissue, inflammation and immunity. Nat Rev Immunol 2006;6:772–83.
57. Spadaro L, Magliocco O, Spampinato D, et al. Effects of n-3 polyunsaturated fatty acids in subjects with nonalcoholic fatty liver disease. Dig Liver Dis 2008;40:194–9.
58. Zhu FS, Liu S, Chen XM, et al. Effects of n-3 polyunsaturated fatty acids from seal oils on nonalcoholic fatty liver disease associated with hyperlipidemia. World J Gastroenterol 2008;14:6395–400.

59. Di Minno MN, Russolillo A, Lupoli R, et al. Omega-3 fatty acids for the treatment of non-alcoholic fatty liver disease. World J Gastroenterol 2012;18:5839–47.
60. Ferruzzi MG. The influence of beverage composition on delivery of phenolic compounds from coffee and tea. Physiol Behav 2010;100:33–41.
61. Freedman ND, Everhart JE, Lindsay KL, et al. Coffee intake is associated with lower rates of liver disease progression in chronic hepatitis C. Hepatology 2009;50:1360–9.
62. Bravi F, Bosetti C, Tavini A, et al. Coffee reduces risk for hepatocellular carcinoma: an updated meta-analysis. Clin Gastroenterol Hepatol 2013. [Epub ahead of print].
63. Molloy JW, Calcagno CJ, Williams CD, et al. Association of coffee and caffeine consumption with fatty liver disease, nonalcoholic steatohepatitis, and degree of hepatic fibrosis. Hepatology 2012;55:429–36.
64. Anty R, Marjoux S, Iannelli A, et al. Regular coffee but no espresso drinking is protective against fibrosis in a cohort mainly composed of morbidly obese European women with NAFLD undergoing bariatric surgery. J Hepatol 2012;57:1090–6.
65. Torres DM, Harrison SA. Is it time to write a prescription for coffee? Coffee and liver disease. Gastroenterology 2013;144:670–2.
66. Mathurin P, Hollebecque A, Arnalsteen L, et al. Prospective study of the long-term effects of bariatric surgery on liver injury in patients without advanced disease. Gastroenterology 2009;137:532–40.
67. Moretto M, Kupski C, da Silva VD, et al. Effect of bariatric surgery on liver fibrosis. Obes Surg 2012;22(7):1044–9.
68. Chavez-Tapia NC, Tellez-Avili FI, Barrientos-Gutierrez T, et al. Bariatric surgery for nonalcoholic steatohepatitis in obese patients. Cochrane Database Syst Rev 2010;(1):CD007340.
69. Zelber-Sagi S, Kessler A, Brazowsky E, et al. A double-blind randomized placebo controlled trial of orlistat for treatment of nonalcoholic fatty liver disease. Clin Gastroenterol Hepatol 2006;4:639–44.
70. Harrison SA, Brunt EM, Fecht WJ, et al. Orlistat for overweight subjects with nonalcoholic steatohepatitis (NASH): a randomized prospective trial. Hepatology 2009;49:80–6.
71. Barkeling B, Elfhag K, Rooth P, et al. Short-term effects of sibutramine (Reductil) on appetite and eating behaviour and the long-term therapeutic outcome. Int J Obes Relat Metab Disord 2003;27:693–700.
72. Sabuncu T, Nazligul Y, Karaoglanoglu M, et al. The effects of sibutramine and orlistat on the ultrasonographic findings, insulin resistance and liver enzyme levels in obese patients with non-alcoholic steatohepatitis. Rom J Gastroenterol 2003;12:189–92.
73. Tziomalo K, Krassas G, Tzotzas T. The use of sibutramine in the management of obesity and related disorders: an update. Vasc Health Risk Manag 2009;5:441–52.
74. James WP, Caterson ID, Coutinho W, et al. Effect of sibutramine on cardiovascular outcomes in overweight and obese subjects. N Engl J Med 2010;363:905–17.
75. Di Dalmazi G, Vicennti V, Pasquali R, et al. The unrelenting fall of the pharmacological treatment of obesity. Endocrine 2013. [Epub ahead of print].
76. Vernon G, Baranova A, Younossi ZM. Systemic review: the epidemiology and natural history of non-alcoholic fatty liver disease and nonalcoholic steatohepatitis in adults. Aliment Pharmacol Ther 2001;34:274–85.

77. Neuschwander-Tetri BA, Brunt EM, Wehmeier KR, et al. Improved nonalcoholic steatohepatitis after 48 weeks of treatment with the PPAR-gamma ligand rosiglitazone. Hepatology 2003;38:1008–17.
78. Promrat K, Lutchman G, Uwaifo GI, et al. A pilot study of pioglitazone treatment for nonalcoholic steatohepatitis. Hepatology 2004;39:188–96.
79. Caldwell SH, Hespenheide EE, Redick JA, et al. A pilot study of a thiazolidinedione, troglitazone, in nonalcoholic steatohepatitis. Am J Gastroenterol 2001;96: 519–25.
80. Sanyal AJ, Mofrad PS, Contos MJ, et al. A pilot study of vitamin E versus vitamin E and pioglitazone for the treatment of nonalcoholic steatohepatitis. Clin Gastroenterol Hepatol 2004;2:1107–15.
81. Ratzui V, Caldwell S, Neuschwander-Tetri BA. Therapeutic trials in nonalcoholic steatohepatitis: insulin sensitizers and related methodological issues. Hepatology 2010;52:2206–15.
82. Belfort R, Harrison SA, Brown K, et al. A placebo-controlled trial of pioglitazone in subjects with nonalcoholic steatohepatitis. N Engl J Med 2006;355: 2297–307.
83. Ratziu V, Giral P, Jacqueminet S, et al. Rosiglitazone for nonalcoholic steatohepatitis: one-year results of the randomized placebo-controlled Fatty Liver Improvement with Rosiglitazone Therapy (FLIRT) Trial. Gastroenterology 2008; 135:100–10.
84. Aithal GP, Thomas JA, Kaye PV, et al. Randomized, placebo-controlled trial of pioglitazone in nondiabetic subjects with nonalcoholic steatohepatitis. Gastroenterology 2008;135:1176–84.
85. Sanyal AJ, Chalasani N, Kowdley KV, et al. Pioglitazone, vitamin E, or placebo for nonalcoholic steatohepatitis. N Engl J Med 2010;362:1675–85.
86. Carious B, Zair Y, Staels B, et al. Effects of the new dual PPAR alpha/delta agonist GFT505 on lipid and glucose homeostasis in abdominal obese patients with combined dyslipidemia or impaired glucose metabolism. Diabetes Care 2011;34:2008–14.
87. Nakajima K. Multidisciplinary pharmacotherapeutic options for nonalcoholic fatty liver disease. Int J Hepatol 2012;2012:950693.
88. Tushuizen ME, Bunick MC, Pouwels PJ, et al. Incretin mimetics as a novel therapeutic option for hepatic steatosis. Liver Int 2006;26:1015–7.
89. Kenny PR, Brady DE, Torres DM, et al. Exenatide in the treatment of diabetic patients with nonalcoholic fatty steatohepatitis: a case-series. Am J Gastroenterol 2010;105:2707–9.
90. Nseir W, Mograbi J, Ghali M. Lipid-lowering agents in nonalcoholic fatty liver disease and steatohepatitis: human studies. Dig Dis Sci 2012;57:1773–81.
91. Gomez-Dominguez E, Gisbert JP, Morento-Monteagudo JA, et al. A pilot study of atorvastatin treatment in dysplipidemic, nonalcoholic fatty liver disease patients. Aliment Pharmacol Ther 2006;23:1643–7.
92. Hyogo H, Ikegami T, Tokushige K, et al. Efficacy of pitavastatin for the treatment of nonalcoholic steatohepatitis with dyslipidemia: an open-label, pilot study. Hepatol Res 2011;41:1057–65.
93. Harrison SA, Torgerson S, Havashi P, et al. Vitamin E and vitamin C treatment improves fibrosis in patients with nonalcoholic steatohepatitis. Am J Gastroenterol 2003;98:2485–90.
94. Miller ER III, Pastor-Barriuso R, Dalal D, et al. Meta-analysis: high dose vitamin E supplementation may increase all cause mortality. Ann Intern Med 2005;142: 37–46.

95. Klein EA, Thompson IM, Tangen CM, et al. Vitamin E and the risk of prostate cancer. The selenium and vitamin E cancer prevention trial (SELECT). JAMA 2011;306:1549–56.

96. Kwon do Y, Jung YS, Kim SJ, et al. Impaired sulfur-amino acid metabolism and oxidative stress in nonalcoholic fatty liver are alleviated by betaine supplementation in rats. J Nutr 2009;139:63–8.

97. Abdelmalek MF, Sanderson SO, Angulo P, et al. Betaine for nonalcoholic steatohepatitis: results of a randomized placebo controlled trial. Heaptology 2009;50: 1818–26.

98. Mazo DF, de Oliveira MG, Pereira IV, et al. S-nitroso-N-acetylcysteine attenuates liver fibrosis in experimental nonalcoholic steatohepatitis. Drug Des Devel Ther 2013;7:553–63.

99. Pamuk GE, Sonsuz A. N-acetylcysteine in the treatment of non-alcoholic steatohepatitis. J Gastroenterol Hepatol 2003;18:1220–1.

100. Khoshbaten M, Aliasgarzadeh A, Masnadi K, et al. N-acetylcysteine improves liver function in patients with non-alcoholic fatty liver disease. Hepat Mon 2010;10:12–6.

101. Laurin J, Lindor KD, Crippin JS, et al. Ursodeoxycholic acid or clofibrate in the treatment of non-alcoholic induced steatohepatitis: a pilot study. Hepatology 1996;23:1464–7.

102. Ratziu V, de Ledinghen V, Oberti F, et al. A randomized control trial of high dose ursodeoxycholic acid for non-alcoholic steatohepatitis. J Hepatol 2011;54: 1011–9.

103. Lindor KD, Kowdley KV, Heathcote EJ, et al. Ursodeoxycholic acid for treatment of nonalcoholic steatohepatitis: results of a randomized trial. Hepatology 2004; 39:770–8.

104. Adams LA, Zein CO, Angulo P, et al. A pilot trial of pentoxifylline in nonalcoholic steatohepatitis. Am J Gastroenterol 2004;99:2365–8.

105. Satapathy SK, Sakhuja P, Malhotra V, et al. Beneficial effects of pentoxifylline on hepatic steatosis, fibrosis, and necroinflammation in patients with non-alcoholic steatohepatitis. J Gastroenterol Hepatol 2006;22:634–8.

106. Zein CO, Verian LM, Gogate P, et al. Pentoxifylline improves nonalcoholic steatohepatitis: a randomized placebo-controlled trial. Hepatology 2011;54:1610–9.

107. Li Z, Yang S, Lin H, et al. Probiotics and antibiotics to TNF inhibit inflammatory activity and improve nonalcoholic fatty liver disease. Hepatology 2003;37:343–50.

108. Loguerrcio C, Federico A, Tuccillo C, et al. Beneficial effects of a probiotic VSL#3 on parameters of liver dysfunction in chronic liver diseases. J Clin Gastroenterol 2005;39:540–3.

109. Hirose A, Ono M, Saibara T, et al. Angiotension II type 1 receptor blocker inhibits fibrosis in rat nonalcoholic steatohepatitis. Hepatology 2007;45:1375–81.

110. Torres DM, Jones FJ, Shaw JC, et al. Rosiglitazone versus rosiglitazone and metformin versus rosiglitazone and losartan in the treatment of nonalcoholic steatohepatitis: a 12-month, randomized, prospective, open-label trial. Hepatology 2011;54:1631–9.

111. Adorini L, Pruzandski M, Shapiro D. Farnesoid X receptor targeting to treat nonalcoholic steatohepatitis. Drug Discov Today 2012;17:988–97.

112. Mudaliar S, Henry RR, Sanyal AJ, et al. Efficacy and safety of the farnesoid X receptor agonist obeticholic acid in patients with type 2 diabetes and nonalcoholic fatty liver disease. Gastroenterology 2013;145:574–82.e1.

Cholestatic Liver Disease

Andrea A. Gossard, MS, CNP*, Jayant A. Talwalkar, MD, MPH

KEYWORDS

- Cholestasis • Biliary tract disease • Bile duct obstruction • Primary biliary cirrhosis
- Primary sclerosing cholangitis • Cholestatic liver disease

KEY POINTS

- Cholestasis may be identified through blood work or may be clinically evident.
- Causes of cholestasis require a thorough review of the patient's medical and surgical history, medication list, and symptomatology.
- Initial evaluation of the cholestatic patient should include imaging of the liver and biliary tree.
- Management of reversible conditions may require endoscopic or surgical intervention.
- Chronic cholestatic liver disease may contribute to fatigue, pruritus, fat-soluble vitamin deficiencies, and bone loss.

INTRODUCTION

Cholestatic liver disease may involve both extrahepatic and intrahepatic bile ducts, or may be limited to one or the other. Cholestasis may be due primary bile duct disease or secondary causes such as stones or tumors. Care of the patient with cholestasis depends on identifying the probable cause, initiating appropriate treatment or intervention, and the recognition and management of potential complications.

DIAGNOSIS AND MANAGEMENT

Symptoms

Patients with cholestatic liver disease may present with pruritus, fatigue, jaundice, dark urine, and/or acholic stools. Many patients; however, are entirely asymptomatic and are diagnosed with cholestatic liver disease only after the incidental discovery of liver test abnormalities on blood work.

Cholestatic patients may present with conjugated hyperbilirubinemia. In fact, extrahepatic biliary obstruction will cause conjugated hyperbilirubinemia in 80% of patients.

Cholestatic Liver Disease Study Group, Division of Gastroenterology and Hepatology, Mayo Clinic, 200 First Street SW, Rochester, MN, USA
* Corresponding author.
E-mail address: Gossard.andrea@mayo.edu

Med Clin N Am 98 (2014) 73–85
http://dx.doi.org/10.1016/j.mcna.2013.09.002
0025-7125/14/$ – see front matter © 2014 Elsevier Inc. All rights reserved.

Cholestasis is considered chronic when present for longer than 6 months. It may be further defined as primarily intrahepatic or extrahepatic, and many cases are acute on chronic. Most chronic cases of cholestasis are intrahepatic, and approximately 50% of these patients will demonstrate conjugated hyperbilirubinemia.

Diagnosis

Clinically, a cholestatic disorder can often be differentiated from a primarily hepatocellular disorder by the liver enzyme pattern. If there is a proportionally greater elevation in the alkaline phosphatase when compared with the aminotransferases, the profile is more consistent with cholestasis. If alkaline phosphatase is elevated in isolation, isoenzyme fractionation may be warranted. The level of γ–glutamyltranspeptidase (GGT) is also often elevated in cholestasis. Serum bile acids are the most sensitive test for cholestasis, but testing is usually not readily available in the clinical setting.

A history of fever, especially when accompanied by rigors or right upper quadrant abdominal pain, is more suggestive of cholangitis, owing to obstructive processes such as choledocholithiasis. These symptoms may be seen in alcoholic disease and, rarely, in the setting of viral hepatitis.[1] Recent surgery in the region of the biliary system may have resulted in an inadvertent injury to a bile duct, and should also be considered as a possible cause.

Abdominal ultrasonography (US) is often the initial imaging performed when evaluating cholestasis. The advantages of US include its relatively low cost, noninvasiveness, and the absence of radiation. US can effectively evaluate for intrahepatic and extrahepatic bile duct dilation and the presence of mass lesions; however, operator variability can be an issue. In addition, technical limitations include the inability to penetrate bone, limitations associated with obesity, and bowel gas obstructing the view. US can differentiate between intrahepatic and extrahepatic causes of biliary tract disease, and can readily identify gallbladder abnormality.[2]

Computed tomography (CT) is less operator dependent than US, is more effective when imaging obese patients, and is less susceptible to obscuring bowel gas when evaluating the distal bile ducts. CT is more accurate than US at identifying the level (88%–97% vs 23%–95%) and the cause (70%–94% vs 38%–94%) of biliary obstruction if present.[3] Disadvantages of CT include its decreased ability to identify choledocholithiasis, and exposure of the patient to radiation.[4]

Magnetic resonance imaging (MRI) is useful in the distinguishing chronic from acute etiology of cholestasis. Use of magnetic resonance cholangiopancreatography (MRCP) is considered a safe, noninvasive tool for evaluating the biliary tree. Advantages include the lack of radiation and sharp contrast resolution between normal and abnormal tissues. The accuracy of MRCP is comparable with that of endoscopic cholangiography. In fact, a review of 67 studies found that for the diagnosis of biliary obstruction, MRCP sensitivity and specificity are 95% and 97%, respectively.[5,6] As the bile ducts are visualized in their normal physiologic state, MRCP may be a better indicator than endoscopic cholangiography of their true caliber. The sensitivity for biliary strictures, however, is lower.[6]

When suspicion is high or signs on cross-sectional imaging suggest mechanical obstruction, direct cholangiography, either endoscopically or percutaneously, may be necessary. The primary advantage of direct cholangiography, such as endoscopic retrograde cholangiopancreatography (ERCP), is the ability to both diagnose and intervene therapeutically when indicated. Unfortunately, 3% to 5% of all patients who undergo ERCP will experience complications such as pancreatitis.[7] Percutaneous transhepatic cholangiography (PTC) should be reserved for patients in whom ERCP is precluded for anatomic reasons.

In certain diseases, such as primary sclerosing cholangitis, cholangiography is essential to making the diagnosis. In the setting of chronic cholestasis detected in middle-aged women with positive antimitochondrial antibodies (AMA), however, cholangiography is seldom needed, as this presentation would point more toward primary biliary cirrhosis.

Many of the conditions in the differential diagnosis may be excluded by history, basic laboratory studies, and imaging studies. A liver biopsy is useful when suspecting unusual conditions such as autoimmune cholangitis or overlap syndromes, or in patients with suspected sarcoidosis.

Differential Diagnosis

The evaluation of cholestasis requires review of potential causes. First, a patient's medication list should be reviewed for possible offending agents. The list of medicines that can cause cholestatic liver injury is extensive and includes estrogens, oral contraceptives, anabolic steroids, phenytoin, cyclosporin, dapsone, and erythromycin (**Box 1**). Use of herbal medicines or teas, vitamins, and other supplements should be reviewed and discontinued when possible. Total parenteral nutrition may also cause cholestasis, but often the specific offending medicine or supplement is not clearly identified.

The most common cause of extrahepatic cholestasis is choledocholithiasis.[8,9] Other causes to consider include extrabiliary tumors, cysts, parasitic infection, and lymphoma (**Box 2**). Extrahepatic causes of chronic cholestatic liver disease should be excluded early because they are potentially reversible, and failure to do so may result in complications such as recurrent cholangitis or secondary biliary cirrhosis.

Box 1
Common drugs that may cause cholestasis
Anabolic steroids and androgens
Amoxicillin–clavulanic acid
Azathioprine
Captopril
Carbamazepine
Chlorpromazine
Chlordiazepoxide
Cyclosporine
Dapsone
Diltiazem
Erythromycin
Gold salts
Imipramine
Nitrofurantoin
Oral contraceptives and estrogen
Phenytoin
5-Fluorouracil or floxuridine

Box 2
Extrahepatic biliary obstruction

Intraductal obstruction/abnormalities

    Gallstones

    Cysts

    Strictures

    Immunoglobulin G4–related disease

    Malignancy of bile ducts

    Malformation

    AIDS cholangiopathy (rare in North America)

    Parasites

Extrinsic compression

    Extrabiliary malignancies

    Pancreatitis

    Lymphoma

Diseases that cause intrahepatic cholestasis include immune-mediated diseases such as primary biliary cirrhosis, primary sclerosing cholangitis, and sarcoidosis (**Box 3**). Hepatocellular diseases that may cause intrahepatic cholestatic liver disease typically include viral hepatitis B, hepatitis C, and alcoholic hepatitis.

Autoimmune hepatitis (AIH) can present similarly to primary biliary cirrhosis (PBC), and some degree of overlap is not uncommon.[10] The precise prevalence is unknown, but perhaps 10% of patients could be classified as having AIH/PBC overlap.[11–13] The majority of patients with autoimmune hepatitis have serum antinuclear and anti–smooth muscle antibodies; however, histologically there is rarely destruction of the

---

Box 3
Intrahepatic cholestasis

Primary biliary cirrhosis

Primary sclerosing cholangitis

Hepatocellular disease

    Alcoholic hepatitis

    Hepatitis B

    Hepatitis C

    Autoimmune hepatitis

Miscellaneous causes

    Sarcoidosis

    Idiopathic adult ductopenia

    Benign recurrent intrahepatic cholestasis

    Cystic fibrosis

    Drug-induced cholestasis

bile ducts. In some cases, differentiating between AIH and PBC is difficult, but under these circumstances patients with AIH will experience a dramatic response to immunosuppressive therapy whereas PBC patients will not.

Chronic cholestatic sarcoidosis, a disease most common in young African American men, can present with features that are histologically similar to PBC and, in some cases, primary sclerosing cholangitis (PSC). Granulomatous destruction of small bile ducts is the hallmark of this condition. The granulomas are typically large and well defined, in contrast to the small and poorly defined granulomas seen in PBC. Most of these patients have hilar adenopathy on chest roentgenograms and other features of sarcoidosis, and do not have AMA.

Benign familial recurrent cholestasis (BRIC) is a rare genetic disorder characterized by recurrent attacks of pruritus and jaundice. During the attack, the levels of serum alkaline phosphatase are elevated. Cholestasis is noted histologically and the cholangiogram is normal. There are 2 unique types of presentation. Mutations in the *ATP8B1* gene cause benign recurrent intrahepatic cholestasis type 1 (BRIC1), and mutations in the *ABCB11* gene cause benign recurrent intrahepatic cholestasis type 2 (BRIC2). In the setting of BRIC1, the genetic mutation leads to buildup of bile in the liver cells. The BRIC2 mutation leads to a reduction in the ability to secrete bile salt as a consequence of decreased function of the bile salt export pump. Symptoms associated with each condition are similar. All cases eventually will go into remission. Cirrhosis does not develop, and the prognosis is excellent.[14]

Patients with cystic fibrosis may have neonatal jaundice that resolves, but recurs later in life.[15] Cystic fibrosis related liver disease is thought to be due to impaired secretory function of the biliary epithelium and absent or dysfunctional cystic fibrosis transmembrane conductance regulator (CFTR) protein. This protein is unique to the epithelial cells that line the bile ducts and gallbladder, and contributes to the first stage of ductal secretion. Cholestasis can develop, and may contribute to secondary hepatocyte injury and focal biliary cirrhosis. If this damage is extensive, portal hypertension may develop.[16–18]

The most common cause of chronic intrahepatic cholestatic liver disease in adults is primary biliary cirrhosis.[19] It is estimated that in the United States the prevalence of PBC is approximately 150 to 400 cases per million individuals. The presence of an elevated level of serum immunoglobulin M and AMA (noted in more than 95% of PBC patients) is helpful in making the diagnosis. The specificity of AMA for PBC is 95%.[20] More than 80% of patients with PBC are female. The terms autoimmune cholangitis and AMA-negative PBC have been used for patients who have clinical and histologic features of PBC but are negative for AMA. These patients are generally positive for antinuclear or anti–smooth muscle antibodies. Autoimmune cholangitis and PBC appear to be part of a disease spectrum with very similar clinical and histologic features and a similar response to therapy. Liver biopsy is helpful in confirmation of PBC, but in patients who have prominent cholestatic liver biochemistries and a strongly positive AMA, liver biopsy is usually unnecessary.

PSC is the second most common cause of intrahepatic cholestasis, and is characterized by an inflammatory, fibrotic process that damages both the intrahepatic and extrahepatic bile ducts.[21] The prevalence of primary sclerosing cholangitis is estimated to range from 50 to 70 cases per million individuals. PSC is more common in men, with a 2:1 male to female ratio. The disease is strongly associated with inflammatory bowel disease, with about 80% of PSC patients having concurrent colitis. Approximately 80% of patients with PSC have chronic ulcerative colitis (CUC), 10% have Crohn colitis, and another 10% may have mixed features or indeterminate colitis.[22] The natural history is more variable than that of PBC. Patients may be asymptomatic, but as the disease progresses, complications including dominant biliary duct strictures often develop. Patients with both PSC and CUC are at an increased risk of developing colorectal cancer as well as cholangiocarcinoma.

AMA are typically absent in patients who have PSC. Other antibodies, such as antinuclear antibodies and antineutrophil cytoplasmic antibodies, are frequently found. Bile duct imaging with either magnetic resonance cholangiography or endoscopic retrograde cholangiography is very helpful in confirming the diagnosis of PSC. Classic cholangiographic features of PSC include multifocal stricturing with saccular segmental dilatation causing a beaded appearance.[23] Usually both the intrahepatic and extrahepatic ducts are involved, but up to 20% of patients have only intrahepatic duct disease. Liver biopsy is useful for histologic confirmation and in staging the disease, but is not always necessary.

Occasionally, patients present with histologic features of PSC in the setting of chronic colitis, but have normal cholangiograms. These patients are considered to have small-duct PSC and comprise approximately 5% of all PSC patients.[24] Small-duct PSC may develop into cholangiographically evident disease over time, but the natural history is less well known.

MANAGEMENT
Primary Biliary Cirrhosis

Ursodeoxycholic acid (UDCA) is the main therapy for PBC. At doses of 13 to 15 mg/kg/d, it has been shown to improve both liver biochemistry and transplantation-free survival, particularly in those patients with early-stage disease.[25,26] Treatment with corticosteroids has been evaluated, but concern regarding bone loss in patients predisposed to osteoporosis is valid.[27] Methotrexate was also studied but was found to be ineffective.[28] Moreover, no clear benefit was noted in patients treated with chlorambucil, azathioprine, or silymarin.[29–31]

Primary Sclerosing Cholangitis

Unfortunately, there is no effective therapy for PSC. UDCA is the most studied, but its role remains unclear with regard to its ability to slow the progression of disease.[32–37] Lindor and colleagues[37] revealed that use of high-dose UDCA (28–30 mg/kg/d) was found to increase the risk of esophageal varices and the need for liver transplantation.[38] Therefore, its use cannot be recommended.

Patients with PSC are at risk for biliary obstruction secondary to strictures. These conditions may be managed endoscopically with balloon dilatation. Biliary stenting may also be performed, but is not clearly superior to balloon dilatation.[39]

Pruritus

The most problematic symptom of cholestasis is pruritus. The etiology remains poorly understood, but may be due to the accumulation of hydrophobic bile acids or endogenous opioids. In the absence of bile duct obstruction amenable to treatment, management of pruritus typically involves oral therapies (**Box 4**). Topical treatments are less helpful.

Cholestyramine at doses of 4 g twice daily is considered the first-line therapy for pruritus.[40] Cholestyramine will improve itching in 80% of cholestatic patients, but palatability can be an issue. In this case colestipol, 15 g twice daily, may be a more tolerable substitute. If deemed ineffective or not well tolerated by the patient, use of rifampin, typically at doses of 150 to 300 mg twice daily, can be considered.[41–44] Rifampin is effective in approximately 50% of patients. Patients should be monitored

| Box 4 |
| Management of pruritus |
| Cholestyramine 4 g twice daily |
| Rifampin 150 to 300 mg twice daily |
| Naltrexone 50 mg per day or nalmefene, 4 to 240 mg per day |
| Sertraline 75 to 100 mg per day |

for rare complications including hepatitis, hemolytic anemia, and renal dysfunction. In case series, drug-induced hepatic dysfunction has been reported in up to 12% of cholestatic patients.[45]

Opioid antagonists, such as naltrexone, are important mediators of itch and have been studied as treatment for cholestatic pruritus.[46–51] Naltrexone may be used at a dose of 50 mg/d, or nalmefene at 4 to 240 mg/d. Problems with opiate withdrawal–type reactions have been noted, however, and this risk should be reviewed with the patient.

There is also evidence to support the use of sertraline, 75 to 100 mg/d, as therapy for pruritus, although many clinicians experience disappointing results with this choice.[52] Initial studies of ondansetron demonstrated efficacy; however, subsequent placebo-controlled evidence suggested no benefit.[53,54] The use of gabapentin has been beneficial in anecdotal cases, but data are limited.

Fatigue

Fatigue is a complex and potentially debilitating symptom associated with cholestatic liver disease. Studies of patients with PBC have found that fatigue is present in 68% to 81% of patients,[55–60] and it is nearly as prevalent in patients with PSC or drug-induced cholestasis.[57,61,62] The pathogenesis of fatigue in cholestasis is not well understood. It seems to involve changes in central neurotransmission, which result from signaling between the diseased liver and the brain.[63] There is poor correlation between the degree of fatigue and the stage of cholestatic disease.

The initial step in managing fatigue is ruling out potentially contributing factors such as depression, anemia, thyroid dysfunction, renal dysfunction, and sleep disturbances. Management options for fatigue are limited, and no therapies have been identified as being clearly beneficial. In PBC, fluoxetine was studied and was not helpful.[64] Modafinil has also been evaluated and may provide benefit, but needs further study.[65,66] Emphasis on stress reduction, healthy lifestyle, avoidance of alcohol and caffeine, regular exercise, and adequate sleep may help.[67,68]

Osteoporosis

Osteoporosis develops in patients with cirrhosis of all causes.[69] Both increased resorption and decreased formation of bone contribute to the development of osteoporosis in cholestatic patients.[70] Screening for bone loss in PBC should be performed with bone mineral density assessment (dual-energy x-ray absorptiometry) at baseline with follow-up at between 1 and 5 years, depending on outcome and general risk of osteoporosis.[71]

Use of calcium, 600 mg twice daily with 400 IU of vitamin D and weight-bearing activities, should be considered as initial treatment, although this does not reliably improve bone density in patients with PBC.[72] Hormone replacement therapy has been shown to improve bone mass in postmenopausal patients with PBC, but the risks associated with this therapy should be reviewed.[73,74] Use of testosterone is not recommended.

Bisphosphonate therapy has proved to be beneficial in patients with PBC and osteoporosis, and should be considered in those patients with significant or progressive bone loss.[75–77] Use of oral bisphosphonate in the setting of esophageal varices, however, is not advised.

Vitamin Deficiency

Patients with cholestatic liver disease rarely present with fat-soluble vitamin deficiencies. In a randomized, placebo-controlled trial of 180 patients with PBC, the proportion of patients with vitamin A, D, E, and K deficiencies was 33.5%, 13.2%, 1.9%, and 7.8% respectively.[78] Patients with chronic cholestatic liver disease are at increased risk for fat-soluble vitamin deficiencies and malabsorption of nutrients, because of the decreased availability of bile salts necessary for absorption in the intestinal lumen.

In the presence of advanced-stage disease, evaluation for vitamin D deficiency should be performed annually. When encountered, 50,000 units of water-soluble vitamin D given once or twice per week are usually sufficient to correct the deficiency. Vitamin A deficiency is uncommon, and may present clinically with night blindness. Vitamin A levels can be measured and when low, replacement with 25,000 to 50,000 units 2 to 3 times per week should be instituted, starting at the lower levels. The adequacy of replacement therapy should be assessed by repeat serum assays because excessive vitamin A has been associated with hepatotoxicity. Vitamin E deficiency has been reported in a few cases of PBC. Typically, vitamin E deficiency causes a neurologic abnormality primarily affecting the posterior columns, characterized by areflexia or loss of proprioception and ataxia. Replacement of vitamin E in these patients has been disappointing; however, patients with low serum levels of vitamin E should be started on replacement therapy, usually 100 mg twice daily.

Celiac sprue has been reported in patients with PBC and PSC. Furthermore, because of the association of PBC with scleroderma, wide-mouth diverticula and bacterial overgrowth seen in scleroderma can complicate PBC. In addition, both PBC and PSC have been associated with pancreatic insufficiency, and this must be considered when dealing with patients who have either of these 2 disorders and evidence of malabsorption.

Dyslipidemia

Approximately 75% of patients with PBC have a total cholesterol level higher than 200 mg/dL. A cross-sectional study showed that patients with early-stage PBC histologically tend to have low levels of low-density lipoproteins (LDL) and marked increases in high-density lipoproteins (HDL). When the disease is advanced, patients are more likely to have marked elevations of LDL with the presence of lipoprotein-X and a significant decrease in HDL.[79] For patients with cholesterol deposits in the form of xanthomas or xanthelasma, therapy with UDCA or cholestyramine may stabilize and even decrease the size of these cutaneous deposits.

Patients with PSC often have lipid levels that are elevated, but there does not seem to be an increased risk of cardiovascular events.[80] The reason for this may be related to the difference in the composition of the LDL. Cholestatic patients have elevated levels of lipoprotein-X, which may actually be protective against atherogenesis.

Portal Hypertension

Varices can develop in persons with cholestatic liver disease as with other forms of liver disease, and are associated with an impaired prognosis.[81,82] Standard screening, prophylaxis, and treatment of varices should be used as with other liver diseases.[83–85] First-line therapy for small varices is typically nonselective β-blockade. If large varices with high-risk stigmata are noted, variceal band ligation may be indicated.

Malignancy

The risk of hepatocellular carcinoma (HCC) and cholangiocarcinoma (CCA) are increased in the setting of chronic cholestatic liver disease. The risk of HCC in PBC is increased particularly in men of advanced age and those with evidence of portal hypertension.[86] Surveillance for malignant transformation in the setting of chronic liver disease should be performed every 6 to 12 months with US or MRI. Use of CT for routine surveillance is not advised, given the potential for excess exposure to radiation. If worrisome findings are noted, interventions such as radiofrequency ablation, alcohol injection, chemoembolization, and orthotopic liver transplantation may increase survival.[87]

The cumulative lifetime risk of cholangiocarcinoma (CCA) in PSC is 10% to 15%[88] Up to 50% of CCA is diagnosed within the first year of PSC diagnosis, after which the yearly incidence is 0.5% to 1.5%. Ongoing surveillance for malignant transformation with serial imaging is recommended.

SUMMARY

The care of the patient with cholestasis hinges on identifying the etiology, treating reversible causes, and managing chronic cholestatic processes. PBC and PSC are important causes of chronic cholestasis, and are the most common causes of cholestatic liver disease. Effective therapy is available for patients with PBC, whereas none exists for patients with PSC. Awareness of the complications that may be associated with cholestasis and implementing the appropriate management are essential.

REFERENCES

1. Heathcote EJ. Diagnosis and management of cholestatic liver disease. Clin Gastroenterol Hepatol 2007;5(7):776–82.
2. Bennett WF, Bova JG. Review of hepatic imaging and a problem-oriented approach to liver masses. Hepatology 1990;12(4 Pt 1):761–75.
3. Reddy SI, Grace ND. Liver imaging. A hepatologist's perspective. Clin Liver Dis 2002;6(1):297–310, ix.
4. Saini S. Imaging of the hepatobiliary tract. N Engl J Med 1997;336(26):1889–94.
5. Romagnuolo J, Bardou M, Rahme E, et al. Magnetic resonance cholangiopancreatography: a meta-analysis of test performance in suspected biliary disease. Ann Intern Med 2003;139(7):547–57.
6. Varghese JC, Liddell RP, Farrell MA, et al. The diagnostic accuracy of magnetic resonance cholangiopancreatography and ultrasound compared with direct cholangiography in the detection of choledocholithiasis. Clin Radiol 1999; 54(9):604–14.
7. Freeman ML, Nelson DB, Sherman S, et al. Complications of endoscopic biliary sphincterotomy. N Engl J Med 1996;335(13):909–18.
8. Mark DH, Flamm CR, Aronson N. Evidence-based assessment of diagnostic modalities for common bile duct stones. Gastrointest Endosc 2002;56(Suppl 6):S190–4.
9. Baillie J, Paulson EK, Vitellas KM. Biliary imaging: a review. Gastroenterology 2003;124(6):1686–99.

10. Heathcote EJ. Overlap of autoimmune hepatitis and primary biliary cirrhosis: an evaluation of a modified scoring system. Am J Gastroenterol 2002;97(5):1090–2.
11. Poupon R, Chazouilleres O, Corpechot C, et al. Development of autoimmune hepatitis in patients with typical primary biliary cirrhosis. Hepatology 2006; 44(1):85–90.
12. Rust C, Beuers U. Overlap syndromes among autoimmune liver diseases. World J Gastroenterol 2008;14(21):3368–73.
13. Czaja AJ. The variant forms of autoimmune hepatitis. Ann Intern Med 1996; 125(7):588–98.
14. Nakamuta M, Sakamoto S, Miyata Y, et al. Benign recurrent intrahepatic cholestasis: a long-term follow-up. Hepatogastroenterology 1994;41(3):287–9.
15. Colombo C, Battezzati PM, Crosignani A, et al. Liver disease in cystic fibrosis: a prospective study on incidence, risk factors, and outcome. Hepatology 2002; 36(6):1374–82.
16. Lindblad A, Glaumann H, Strandvik B. Natural history of liver disease in cystic fibrosis. Hepatology 1999;30(5):1151–8.
17. Efrati O, Barak A, Modan-Moses D, et al. Liver cirrhosis and portal hypertension in cystic fibrosis. Eur J Gastroenterol Hepatol 2003;15(10):1073–8.
18. Colombo C, Crosignani A, Battezzati PM. Liver involvement in cystic fibrosis [review]. J Hepatol 1999;31(5):946–54.
19. Ludwig J. Idiopathic adulthood ductopenia: an update. Mayo Clin Proc 1998; 73(3):285–91.
20. Invernizzi P, Lleo A, Podda M. Interpreting serological tests in diagnosing autoimmune liver diseases. Semin Liver Dis 2007;27(2):161–72.
21. Maggs JR, Chapman RW. An update on primary sclerosing cholangitis. Curr Opin Gastroenterol 2008;24(3):377–83.
22. Loftus EV Jr, Harewood GC, Loftus CG, et al. PSC-IBD: a unique form of inflammatory bowel disease associated with primary sclerosing cholangitis. Gut 2005; 54(1):91–6.
23. MacCarty RL, LaRusso NF, Wiesner RH, et al. Primary sclerosing cholangitis: findings on cholangiography and pancreatography. Radiology 1983;149(1): 39–44.
24. Bjornsson E, Olsson R, Bergquist A, et al. The natural history of small-duct primary sclerosing cholangitis. Gastroenterology 2008;134(4):975–80.
25. Lindor KD, Poupon R, Heathcote EJ, et al. Ursodeoxycholic acid for primary biliary cirrhosis. Lancet 2000;355(9204):657–8.
26. Corpechot C, Carrat F, Bahr A, et al. The effect of ursodeoxycholic acid therapy on the natural course of primary biliary cirrhosis. Gastroenterology 2005;128(2): 297–303.
27. Mitchison HC, Palmer JM, Bassendine MF, et al. A controlled trial of prednisolone treatment in primary biliary cirrhosis. Three-year results. J Hepatol 1992; 15(3):336–44.
28. Hendrickse MT, Rigney E, Giaffer MH, et al. Low-dose methotrexate is ineffective in primary biliary cirrhosis: long-term results of a placebo-controlled trial. Gastroenterology 1999;117(2):400–7.
29. Angulo P, Patel T, Jorgensen RA, et al. Silymarin in the treatment of patients with primary biliary cirrhosis with a suboptimal response to ursodeoxycholic acid. Hepatology 2000;32(5):897–900.
30. Christensen E, Neuberger J, Crowe J, et al. Beneficial effect of azathioprine and prediction of prognosis in primary biliary cirrhosis. Final results of an international trial. Gastroenterology 1985;89(5):1084–91.

31. Hoofnagle JH, Davis GL, Schafer DF, et al. Randomized trial of chlorambucil for primary biliary cirrhosis. Gastroenterology 1986;91(6):1327–34.
32. Beuers U, Spengler U, Kruis W, et al. Ursodeoxycholic acid for treatment of primary sclerosing cholangitis: a placebo-controlled trial. Hepatology 1992;16(3):707–14.
33. Stiehl A. Ursodeoxycholic acid in the treatment of primary sclerosing cholangitis. Ann Med 1994;26(5):345–9.
34. Lindor KD. Ursodiol for primary sclerosing cholangitis. Mayo Primary Sclerosing Cholangitis-Ursodeoxycholic Acid Study Group. N Engl J Med 1997;336(10):691–5.
35. Cullen SN, Rust C, Fleming K, et al. High dose ursodeoxycholic acid for the treatment of primary sclerosing cholangitis is safe and effective. J Hepatol 2008;48(5):792–800.
36. Olsson R, Boberg KM, de Muckadell OS, et al. High-dose ursodeoxycholic acid in primary sclerosing cholangitis: a 5-year multicenter, randomized, controlled study. Gastroenterology 2005;129(5):1464–72.
37. Lindor KD, Kowdley KV, Luketic VA, et al. High-dose ursodeoxycholic acid for the treatment of primary sclerosing cholangitis. Hepatology 2009;50(3):808–14.
38. Imam MH, Sinakos E, Gossard AA, et al. High-dose ursodeoxycholic acid increases risk of adverse outcomes in patients with early stage primary sclerosing cholangitis. Aliment Pharmacol Ther 2011;34(10):1185–92.
39. Kaya M, Petersen BT, Angulo P, et al. Balloon dilation compared to stenting of dominant strictures in primary sclerosing cholangitis. Am J Gastroenterol 2001;96(4):1059–66.
40. Imam MH, Gossard AA, Sinakos E, et al. Pathogenesis and management of pruritus in cholestatic liver disease. J Gastroenterol Hepatol 2012;27(7):1150–8.
41. Ghent CN, Carruthers SG. Treatment of pruritus in primary biliary cirrhosis with rifampin. Results of a double-blind, crossover, randomized trial. Gastroenterology 1988;94(2):488–93.
42. Heathcote EJ. Is rifampin a safe and effective treatment for pruritus caused by chronic cholestasis? Nat Clin Pract Gastroenterol Hepatol 2007;4(4):200–1.
43. Bachs L, Pares A, Elena M, et al. Effects of long-term rifampicin administration in primary biliary cirrhosis. Gastroenterology 1992;102(6):2077–80.
44. Podesta A, Lopez P, Terg R, et al. Treatment of pruritus of primary biliary cirrhosis with rifampin. Dig Dis Sci 1991;36(2):216–20.
45. Prince MI, Burt AD, Jones DE. Hepatitis and liver dysfunction with rifampicin therapy for pruritus in primary biliary cirrhosis. Gut 2002;50(3):436–9.
46. Heathcote J. The pruritus of cholestasis is relieved by an opiate antagonist: is this pruritus a centrally mediated phenomenon? Hepatology 1996;23(5):1280–2.
47. Bergasa NV, Alling DW, Talbot TL, et al. Oral nalmefene therapy reduces scratching activity due to the pruritus of cholestasis: a controlled study. J Am Acad Dermatol 1999;41(3 Pt 1):431–4.
48. Thornton JR, Losowsky MS. Opioid peptides and primary biliary cirrhosis. BMJ 1988;297(6662):1501–4.
49. Bergasa NV, Alling DW, Talbot TL, et al. Effects of naloxone infusions in patients with the pruritus of cholestasis. A double-blind, randomized, controlled trial. Ann Intern Med 1995;123(3):161–7.
50. Bergasa NV, Jones EA. The pruritus of cholestasis: potential pathogenic and therapeutic implications of opioids. Gastroenterology 1995;108(5):1582–8.
51. Wolfhagen FH, Sternieri E, Hop WC, et al. Oral naltrexone treatment for cholestatic pruritus: a double-blind, placebo-controlled study. Gastroenterology 1997;113(4):1264–9.

52. Mayo MJ, Handem I, Saldana S, et al. Sertraline as a first-line treatment for cholestatic pruritus. Hepatology 2007;45(3):666–74.
53. Muller C, Pongratz S, Pidlich J, et al. Treatment of pruritus in chronic liver disease with the 5-hydroxytryptamine receptor type 3 antagonist ondansetron: a randomized, placebo-controlled, double-blind cross-over trial. Eur J Gastroenterol Hepatol 1998;10(10):865–70.
54. O'Donohue JW, Pereira SP, Ashdown AC, et al. A controlled trial of ondansetron in the pruritus of cholestasis. Aliment Pharmacol Ther 2005;21(8):1041–5.
55. Witt-Sullivan H, Heathcote J, Cauch K, et al. The demography of primary biliary cirrhosis in Ontario, Canada. Hepatology 1990;12(1):98–105.
56. Cauch-Dudek K, Abbey S, Stewart DE, et al. Fatigue in primary biliary cirrhosis. Gut 1998;43(5):705–10.
57. Huet PM, Deslauriers J, Tran A, et al. Impact of fatigue on the quality of life of patients with primary biliary cirrhosis. Am J Gastroenterol 2000;95(3):760–7.
58. Vuoristo M, Farkkila M, Karvonen AL, et al. A placebo-controlled trial of primary biliary cirrhosis treatment with colchicine and ursodeoxycholic acid. Gastroenterology 1995;108(5):1470–8.
59. Lindor KD, Dickson ER, Baldus WP, et al. Ursodeoxycholic acid in the treatment of primary biliary cirrhosis. Gastroenterology 1994;106(5):1284–90.
60. Heathcote EJ, Cauch-Dudek K, Walker V, et al. The Canadian multicenter double-blind randomized controlled trial of ursodeoxycholic acid in primary biliary cirrhosis. Hepatology 1994;19(5):1149–56.
61. Gross CR, Malinchoc M, Kim WR, et al. Quality of life before and after liver transplantation for cholestatic liver disease. Hepatology 1999;29(2):356–64.
62. Katsinelos P, Vasiliadis T, Xiarchos P, et al. Ursodeoxycholic acid (UDCA) for the treatment of amoxicillin-clavulanate potassium (Augmentin)-induced intrahepatic cholestasis: report of two cases. Eur J Gastroenterol Hepatol 2000; 12(3):365–8.
63. Swain MG. Fatigue in liver disease: pathophysiology and clinical management. Can J Gastroenterol 2006;20(3):181–8.
64. Talwalkar JA, Donlinger JJ, Gossard AA, et al. Fluoxetine for the treatment of fatigue in primary biliary cirrhosis: a randomized, double-blind controlled trial. Dig Dis Sci 2006;51(11):1985–91.
65. Abbas G, Jorgensen RA, Lindor KD. Fatigue in primary biliary cirrhosis. Nat Rev Gastroenterol Hepatol 2010;7(6):313–9.
66. Ian Gan S, de Jongh M, Kaplan MM. Modafinil in the treatment of debilitating fatigue in primary biliary cirrhosis: a clinical experience. Dig Dis Sci 2009; 54(10):2242–6.
67. Swain MG. Fatigue in chronic disease. Clin Sci (Lond) 2000;99(1):1–8.
68. Bergasa NV, Mehlman JK, Jones EA. Pruritus and fatigue in primary biliary cirrhosis. Baillieres Best Pract Res Clin Gastroenterol 2000;14(4):643–55.
69. Sokhi RP, Anantharaju A, Kondaveeti R, et al. Bone mineral density among cirrhotic patients awaiting liver transplantation. Liver Transpl 2004;10(5):648–53.
70. Guichelaar MM, Malinchoc M, Sibonga J, et al. Bone metabolism in advanced cholestatic liver disease: analysis by bone histomorphometry. Hepatology 2002;36(4 Pt 1):895–903.
71. Newton J, Francis R, Prince M, et al. Osteoporosis in primary biliary cirrhosis revisited. Gut 2001;49(2):282–7.
72. Crippin JS, Jorgensen RA, Dickson ER, et al. Hepatic osteodystrophy in primary biliary cirrhosis: effects of medical treatment. Am J Gastroenterol 1994;89(1): 47–50.

73. Pereira SP, O'Donohue J, Moniz C, et al. Transdermal hormone replacement therapy improves vertebral bone density in primary biliary cirrhosis: results of a 1-year controlled trial. Aliment Pharmacol Ther 2004;19(5):563–70.

74. Boone RH, Cheung AM, Girlan LM, et al. Osteoporosis in primary biliary cirrhosis: a randomized trial of the efficacy and feasibility of estrogen/progestin. Dig Dis Sci 2006;51(6):1103–12.

75. Guanabens N, Pares A, Ros I, et al. Alendronate is more effective than etidronate for increasing bone mass in osteopenic patients with primary biliary cirrhosis. Am J Gastroenterol 2003;98(10):2268–74.

76. Musialik J, Petelenz M, Gonciarz Z. Effects of alendronate on bone mass in patients with primary biliary cirrhosis and osteoporosis: preliminary results after one year. Scand J Gastroenterol 2005;40(7):873–4.

77. Zein CO, Jorgensen RA, Clarke B, et al. Alendronate improves bone mineral density in primary biliary cirrhosis: a randomized placebo-controlled trial. Hepatology 2005;42(4):762–71.

78. Phillips JR, Angulo P, Petterson T, et al. Fat-soluble vitamin levels in patients with primary biliary cirrhosis. Am J Gastroenterol 2001;96(9):2745–50.

79. Jahn CE, Schaefer EJ, Taam LA, et al. Lipoprotein abnormalities in primary biliary cirrhosis. Association with hepatic lipase inhibition as well as altered cholesterol esterification. Gastroenterology 1985;89(6):1266–78.

80. Sinakos E, Abbas G, Jorgensen RA, et al. Serum lipids in primary sclerosing cholangitis. Dig Liver Dis 2012;44(1):44–8.

81. Gores GJ, Wiesner RH, Dickson ER, et al. Prospective evaluation of esophageal varices in primary biliary cirrhosis: development, natural history, and influence on survival. Gastroenterology 1989;96(6):1552–9.

82. Jones DE, Metcalf JV, Collier JD, et al. Hepatocellular carcinoma in primary biliary cirrhosis and its impact on outcomes. Hepatology 1997;26(5):1138–42.

83. Garcia-Tsao G, Sanyal AJ, Grace ND, et al. Prevention and management of gastroesophageal varices and variceal hemorrhage in cirrhosis. Hepatology 2007;46(3):922–38.

84. Bressler B, Pinto R, El-Ashry D, et al. Which patients with primary biliary cirrhosis or primary sclerosing cholangitis should undergo endoscopic screening for oesophageal varices detection? Gut 2005;54(3):407–10.

85. Bruix J, Sherman M. Management of hepatocellular carcinoma. Hepatology 2005;42(5):1208–36.

86. Suzuki A, Lymp J, Donlinger J, et al. Clinical predictors for hepatocellular carcinoma in patients with primary biliary cirrhosis. Clin Gastroenterol Hepatol 2007;5(2):259–64.

87. Imam MH, Silveira MG, Sinakos E, et al. Long-term outcomes of patients with primary biliary cirrhosis and hepatocellular carcinoma. Clin Gastroenterol Hepatol 2012;10(2):182–5.

88. Lazaridis KN, Gores GJ. Primary sclerosing cholangitis and cholangiocarcinoma. Semin Liver Dis 2006;26(1):42–51.

Metal Storage Disorders
Wilson Disease and Hemochromatosis

Pushpjeet Kanwar, MD, Kris V. Kowdley, MD*

KEYWORDS

- Hemochromatosis • Hepcidin • Ferritin • Cirrhosis • Wilson disease • Copper

KEY POINTS

- A diagnosis of hereditary hemochromatosis (HH) usually requires an elevated serum ferritin (SF) and transferrin-iron saturation (TS) with C282Y homozygosity on *HFE* genetic testing.
- C282Y homozygous individuals with an SF level higher than 1000 µg/L have an increased risk of cirrhosis and mortality in comparison with those with an SF level lower than 1000 µg/L.
- A liver biopsy is only required in HH if SF is greater than 1000 µg/L in C282Y homozygotes or if there is suspicion of another liver disease.
- Wilson disease can present as chronic disease, acute liver failure, or acute on chronic liver disease, commonly in young individuals between 5 and 40 years of age.
- A diagnosis of Wilson disease is usually made by a combination of a low serum ceruloplasmin, increased 24-hour urine copper levels, or the presence of a Kayser-Fleischer ring on ophthalmologic slit-lamp examination.
- Liver biopsy is required in uncertain cases, although genetic testing is increasingly replacing its use as a confirmatory study, making histologic evaluation merely a staging study or a means of diagnosing concomitant liver diseases.

INTRODUCTION

Hereditary hemochromatosis (HH) and Wilson disease are metal storage disorders that result in accumulation of iron and copper, respectively, in various organs, primarily the liver. Both diseases have certain similarities such as autosomal recessive

Financial Disclosure: Dr Kowdley has served as a scientific advisor to Novartis, the maker of deferasirox, and has received honoraria payable to his institution; Dr Kanwar has no relevant affiliations or financial involvement with any organization or entity with a financial interest in or financial conflict with the subject matter or materials discussed in the article. No writing assistance was commissioned in the production of this article.
Liver Center of Excellence, Department of Gastroenterology, Digestive Disease Institute, Virginia Mason Medical Center, 1100 9th Avenue, Mailstop C3-GAS, Seattle, WA 98101, USA
* Corresponding author.
E-mail address: Kris.kowdley@vmmc.org

heritability and a variable phenotypic spectrum. A diagnosis can be made in both diseases with genetic testing. There are also significant differences between these disorders. Wilson disease has a much lower incidence, earlier age at onset and presentation, is more likely to present with symptoms, and can present with acute liver failure. By contrast, HH is a chronic disease with later age onset, lower rate of penetrance, fewer symptoms, and an expressivity that depends on multiple genetic and environmental factors. Although iron and copper cause different disorders, they can frequently affect each other's concentration in the human body. Moreover, both metals participate in redox reactions through their oxidation states (Fe^{3+}/Fe^{3+} and Cu^{2+}/Cu^{+}). Excess of these metals can lead to cell injury by oxidative stress and lipid peroxidation, which is responsible for damage to various cellular organelles such as mitochondria, lysosomes, cell membrane, and even the nuclear DNA.[1–5] These metals also work closely with each other. Ceruloplasmin, a protein that binds copper and aids in its biliary excretion, also works as ferroxidase to help utilize tissue iron. Although Wilson disease is associated with low levels of serum ceruloplasmin, a complete lack of this protein leads to an iron overload disorder called aceruloplasminemia.[6]

HEREDITARY HEMOCHROMATOSIS

HH includes a group of disorders in which the central mechanism of action involves lack of appropriate hepcidin response to body iron stores.[7] Hepcidin is a peptide hormone, encoded by a gene expressed in the liver, which controls iron absorption in the duodenum.[8] Hepcidin secretion is increased proportionately to iron absorption in duodenum, similar to the action of insulin in hyperglycemia.[9] Hepcidin prevents cellular iron export by binding to and internalizing ferroportin, which exports iron from cells.[10] The expression of hepcidin is regulated by multiple iron-sensing molecules such as BMP6 and proteins encoded by genes such as *HFE*, transferrin receptor 2 (*TFR2*), *HAMP*, and hemojuvelin (*HJV*). In HH, underlying mutations in any of these genes (or ferroportin gene) leads to a deficient hepcidin response, resulting in uncontrolled efflux of iron from enterocytes and macrophages, and iron overload in liver and other tissues.[8] It is still not clear as to how the *HFE* mutation product controls the hepcidin gene.

The most common type of HH is *HFE*-associated HH (classic or Type 1), which is responsible for most cases. The disease is autosomal recessive and involves mutations in the *HFE* gene on chromosome 6.[11] Approximately 80% to 90% of *HFE*-related HH cases are due to homozygous C282Y mutations,[8,12] whereby cysteine is replaced by tyrosine at position 282. This mutation is almost exclusively (prevalence approximately 1 in 200 to 300) seen in individuals with Northern European ancestry.[8] H63D is another *HFE* mutation associated with HH with a more global prevalence, whereby aspartic acid is substituted for histidine at position 63 of the gene.[13] However, over the last decade it has become apparent that the H63D mutation (homozygous or heterozygous) is not associated with significant iron overload.[14] Usually this is also the case among C282Y/H63D compound heterozygotes, who account for approximately 5% cases of HH and commonly develop iron overload only in the presence of another liver disease.[15,16]

Diagnosis

The diagnosis of HH is usually made by a combination of clinical features, imaging, laboratory tests, and genetic testing. The need for liver biopsy is now becoming less frequent unless a concomitant liver disease is expected or there is suspicion of cirrhosis based on other available clinical data.

Clinical features

Excess iron deposition in various organs because of HH can cause a variety of symptoms and signs (**Table 1**). The predominant organs include liver, heart, gonads, pituitary, pancreas, joints, and skin. Iron overload in these organs can lead to cirrhosis, cardiomyopathy, hypogonadism, hypopituitarism, diabetes mellitus, arthropathy (typically the second or third metacarpophalangeal joints), and bronze skin pigmentation.[16] It is difficult to ascertain the actual clinical penetrance of C282Y homozygous HH because different studies have a different definition of iron-overload–related morbidity. Some have lacked a control population, making it difficult to identify symptoms as being related to iron overload.[17] Nevertheless, the mutation has a low penetrance, and approximately 24% to 43% of males and 1% to 14% of females with C282Y homozygous mutation will express the clinical phenotype.[17] Hepatocellular carcinoma is an important complication and is seen in approximately 6% men and 1.5% women with HH.[18]

Biochemical testing

Serum ferritin (SF) and transferrin-iron saturation (TS) are usually elevated on laboratory testing in patients with HH, and can act as the initial screening test when there is suspicion of HH. The upper limit of normal for SF is 300 µg/L for men and 200 µg/L for women, and 45% for TS.[19,20] Elevation of these indices is frequently the initial reason for further evaluation for HH in a patient. The calculation of TS is performed by dividing serum iron by total iron-binding capacity (TIBC). The likelihood of presence of HH phenotype or even the genotype is extremely low in patients with mild to moderate elevation in SF, but normal TS.[21,22] Similarly, not every patient with the C282Y homozygous genotype will develop abnormal iron indices. Based on 2 large population-based studies in North America and Australia, roughly three-quarters of men and 50% of women with the C282Y homozygous genotype will have elevated SF and TS at baseline.[23,24] The presence of an SF level higher than 1000 µg/L predicts a greater risk of development of clinical symptoms and cirrhosis, and is associated with a higher risk of mortality.[24–26]

Genetic testing

Gene testing for type 1 or *HFE*-associated HH is routinely available, unlike for other rare types of HH. Testing for Hemojuvelin or *HJV* (type 2a HH), hepcidin antimicrobial peptide gene or *HAMP* gene (type 2b HH), transferrin receptor 2 or *TfR2* (type 3HH), and SLC40A1 (type 4 HH or ferroportin disease) is only possible in a few centers in the world.[27] These rare types have been shown to be associated with different types

Table 1		
Clinical features of hereditary hemochromatosis		
Organ	**Symptom or Presentation**	**Sign/End Organ Damage**
Liver	RUQ abdominal pain	Hepatomegaly/cirrhosis
Heart	CHF symptoms	Murmurs/cardiomyopathy
Gonads/pituitary	Impotence, loss of libido	Small testes
Pancreas	Hyperglycemia	Diabetes
Skin	Skin discoloration	Bronze skin pigmentation
Joints	Pain in 2nd/3rd MCP	Boggy, tender joints/arthritis

Abbreviations: CHF, congestive heart failure; MCP, metacarpophalangeal joint; RUQ, right upper quadrant.

of mutations (missense, nonsense, frameshift, or promoter) at different positions of the gene.[28] Ferroportin disease differs from other types, as it is autosomal dominant with generally missense mutations, and is a milder disease with low TS and hypochromic anemia, making phlebotomy problematic.[28]

With the advent of *HFE* testing in 1996, genetic testing has replaced liver biopsy as the confirmatory test in most cases. C282Y homozygotes with elevated iron indices do not need further evaluation with a liver biopsy, and can start treatment. However, if SF is greater than 1000 µg/L, patients will need a liver biopsy to rule out cirrhosis (**Fig. 1**). Patients with other HFE genotypes develop the biochemical or clinical phenotype only in the presence of risk factors (such as excess alcohol intake, viral hepatitis, or fatty liver) for other concomitant liver diseases, and a liver biopsy is helpful in ruling them in or out (**Fig. 2**).[29] C282Y homozygotes without evidence of iron overload can be followed with annual SF measurements.[16]

Hepatic iron concentration

Calculation of hepatic iron concentration (HIC) can be important in cases where the diagnosis of iron overload cannot be made by laboratory or genetic testing. A HIC level of greater than 4000 µg/g dry weight of liver is diagnostic of the HH phenotype. Noninvasively, it is calculated by performing T2* magnetic resonance imaging (MRI) or a Ferriscan (Resonance Health Ltd, Claremont, WA, Australia).[30] These noninvasive tests are preferred over a liver biopsy in cases where SF is less than 1000 µg/L and there is no suspicion of another liver disease. The noninvasive measurement of hepatic iron depends on the paramagnetic properties of iron, which increase the relaxation time of protons. This loss of signal intensity is inversely proportional to the HIC.[30] The calculated HIC has high sensitivity and specificity in predicting iron overload, although it may lack the precision of a liver biopsy.[31]

Liver-biopsy measurement of hepatic iron content has historically been the gold standard, but is more invasive and is limited by sampling variability.[32] Nevertheless, the staining pattern of iron with Perls Prussian blue on a liver biopsy is useful in non-C282Y homozygotes with other concomitant liver diseases. A predominant hepatocellular pattern of 3+ or more iron staining differentiates the HH iron overload from a mixed (hepatocytes and Kupffer cells) or mesenchymal pattern of iron staining seen in other liver diseases such as nonalcoholic steatohepatitis.[33] The usefulness of liver biopsy in evaluating for cirrhosis in patients with SF greater than 1000 µg/L is also

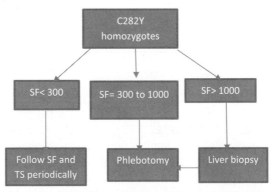

Fig. 1. Diagnostic schema for C282Y homozygotes. SF (serum ferritin) values are in µg/L; liver biopsy should be performed if there is suspicion of another liver disease regardless of SF levels. Upper limit of normal for SF is 200 µg/L in women. TS, transferrin saturation.

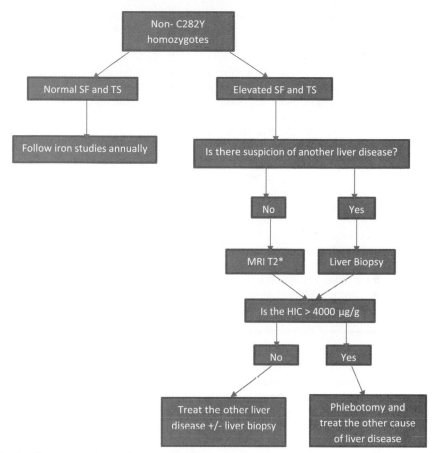

Fig. 2. Diagnostic schema for non-C282Y homozygotes, which include C282Y compound heterozygotes, C282Y heterozygotes, H63D homozygotes, and H63D heterozygotes. Patients with no mutations do not usually need further workup if there is a clear cause of elevated iron indices such as presence of chronic inflammatory diseases (eg, rheumatoid arthritis) or dyserythropoietic anemia, unless the iron indices are significantly elevated. HIC, hepatic iron concentration; SF, serum ferritin; TS, transferrin saturation.

progressively becoming limited as other noninvasive tests such as transient elastography are being increasingly used around the world to stage the liver disease.[34] Other tests such as a combination of hyaluronic acid and SF have also been found to be effective for the prediction of cirrhosis.[35]

Treatment

Therapeutic phlebotomy (venesection) remains the mainstay of treatment for HH patients. Phlebotomy can reverse some of the complications such as fibrosis, skin pigmentation, fatigue, and, rarely, hypogonadism, but joint damage, cirrhosis, diabetes, and cardiomyopathy may not be reversible.[36–39] Iron overloading has been shown to be associated with a variety of cancers, emphasizing iron's possible role in carcinogenesis.[40] This finding supports the hypothesis that iron depletion may be useful in cirrhotic patients and may decrease the risk of hepatocellular carcinoma.

Venesection is also useful in patients with secondary iron overload attributable to other liver diseases such as nonalcoholic steatohepatitis (NASH) and hepatitis C.[29] The treatment goals with phlebotomy are similar for HH and iron overload resulting from these liver diseases.[29]

The goal of therapy is to bring the SF down to normal levels rapidly with weekly removal of one unit (400–500 mL) of blood, which contains 200 to 250 mg iron. However, it is very important to follow the hemoglobin closely, making sure the level does not drop more than 20% of the initial hemoglobin level.[29] The frequency of monitoring SF depends on the initial ferritin. It is usually checked every 10 to 12 phlebotomies; the frequency is decreased when the SF reaches normal levels and is discontinued when SF levels reach 50 to 100 μg/L. Once goal SF levels are reached, the iron indices should be followed periodically to monitor for iron reaccumulation.[29]

The philosophy that all patients with HH should undergo phlebotomy treatment to an SF less than 50 μg/L is changing.[29] Because most otherwise asymptomatic C282Y homozygotes do not develop iron overload disease, as shown by the Health-Iron study,[24] wherein only 28% of men and 1% of women developed iron-overload–related morbidity, expectant management with routine monitoring of SF and TS should be considered for asymptomatic HH patients with normal iron indices.[16] Moreover, even those undergoing phlebotomy do not need to achieve and maintain an SF lower than 50 μg/L, as low iron stores can paradoxically cause a further decrease in hepcidin and may lead to reaccumulation of iron.[41]

Rarely, patients lack compliance with phlebotomy or suffer from hematologic disorders such as thalassemia and, thus, have low baseline hemoglobin, making phlebotomy intolerable. These individuals may benefit from oral iron chelators such as deferasirox at a dose of 10 mg/kg/d, which can decrease SF by 75%.[42] Deferasirox can cause gastrointestinal side effects, kidney damage, and liver toxicity.[42] Erythrocytapheresis is an upcoming treatment whereby red blood cells are selectively removed, thereby decreasing the frequency of treatment visits.[43]

Liver transplantation is a curative treatment option that historically has been known to have poor outcomes in HH patients. However, a recent study showed that post-transplant outcomes are not worse than with other diagnoses.[44] Furthermore, liver transplantation for HH results in normalization of hepcidin levels and prevents iron overload in the transplanted liver.[44]

Survival and Screening

Untreated HH patients with the clinical phenotype or C282Y homozygous genotype have a higher mortality risk in comparison with the general population.[45,46] Cirrhotic patients with HH have a higher mortality risk with and without treatment. Survival of patients without diabetes and cirrhosis is similar to that in the general population if they are adequately iron depleted.[47] Phlebotomy likely improves survival, but there is no prospective study comparing it with placebo, in part because of ethical concerns regarding withholding a proven effective and safe treatment in HH patients.

Screening for HH in the general population has not been shown to be beneficial and is not cost-effective.[19] However, some have advocated for screening for HH using TS in selected populations at higher risk, such as men with northern European ancestry.[48] First-degree relatives of HH individuals should be offered genetic screening and testing of iron indices, whereas children of HH patients do not need genetic screening if the spouse of the HH patient has a wild-type *HFE* genotype.[49] Moreover, children do not need to be offered screening before adulthood because the risk of developing clinical HH before age 18 is negligible.[50]

WILSON DISEASE

Wilson disease is an autosomal recessive disorder with a global incidence considered to be 1 in 30,000.[51] However, a recent study from the United Kingdom suggested that the incidence may be much higher, and closer to 1 in 7000.[52] The pathogenesis involves homozygous mutation in the ATP7B gene,[53–55] which leads to loss of biliary secretion of copper. In turn this leads to overloading of this metal in various organs such as the liver, basal ganglia, and cornea.[56] The disease is named after Dr Samuel Alexander Kinnear Wilson, who published an article (based on a thesis) in the journal *Brain* in March 1912.[57] This article, on "progressive lenticular degeneration," described a neurologic condition associated with cirrhosis seen in a group of patients seen by him and by others previously, including Sir William Gowers.[58]

The primary genetic defect, discovered in 1993, lies in a large 21-exon gene on chromosome 13. The ATP7B gene encodes a 1456-amino-acid protein with 6 copper-binding domains.[59] This "Wilson disease protein" is a P-type adenosine triphosphatase that helps in the transport of copper. Normally, 40% to 60% of dietary copper is absorbed from the proximal small intestine and is directed into the portal circulation with the help of another copper-transporting enzyme produced by the ATP7A gene. Mutations in the *ATP7A* gene lead to a copper-deficiency disease called Menkes disease.[60] Absorbed copper is bound to albumin (free copper) and reaches the liver through the portal vasculature. It is transported into liver cells with the help of a human copper transporter, HCTR1. Subsequently copper enters the hepatocytes and is released into the bile through conjugation with glutathione, but the primary mechanism involves the ATP7B protein. This protein moves copper through the trans-Golgi network and forms vesicles that which fuse with the membranes of the bile canaliculi, following which copper is excreted into the bile after incorporation into ceruloplasmin.[61] Mutations in the *ATP7B* gene lead to accumulation of copper in the liver, leading to cell injury and apoptosis, fibrosis, and, eventually, cirrhosis.[62]

Diagnosis

The diagnosis of Wilson disease is made by a combination of clinical, laboratory, and histologic findings. Genetic testing is usually reserved for uncertain cases and can provide a definitive diagnosis of the genetic abnormality. Most cases are diagnosed with the help of clinical history, physical examination, and laboratory testing of serum and urine (**Fig. 3**). Liver biopsy is usually needed to evaluate hepatic copper concentration and staging of the disease.

Clinical presentation

Patients with Wilson disease have an early onset of disease activity, and usually present with symptoms between 5 and 40 years of age.[56] Liver, brain, and cornea are the most common organs affected. As with other liver diseases, chronic hepatic injury does not cause many symptoms, and the only abnormality usually seen is elevated aminotransferases or hepatomegaly. However, Wilson disease can present as acute liver failure (ALF) with hemolytic anemia, elevated international normalized ratio, and jaundice caused by liver dysfunction and hemolysis. Frequently, ALF caused by Wilson disease is associated with kidney injury, and occasionally patients develop aminoaciduria. Young women may have an increased risk of developing ALF.[63]

Neurologic symptoms are usually late in onset but can be seen in children. These symptoms include dysarthria, dystonia, tremors, ataxia, drooling, speech deficits, autonomic dysfunction, and parkinsonian rigidity.[56,64,65] Some symptoms, such as dystonia and spasticity, can cause significant disability, and the patient can become bed-bound.[56,64] These findings can be confused with those of other neurologic

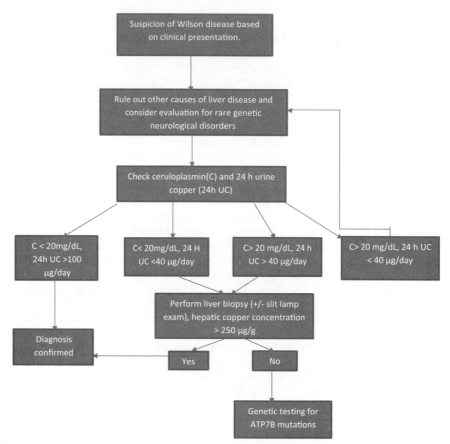

Fig. 3. Diagnostic testing in Wilson disease. Presence of Kayser-Fleischer (KF) rings usually is diagnostic of Wilson disease, although they are usually seen with neurologic presentation of the disease. Slit-lamp examination for evaluation of KF rings can be performed before performing a liver biopsy, whereby only 1 of the laboratory markers (serum ceruloplasmin or 24-hour urine copper) is suggestive of Wilson disease.

disorders and hepatic encephalopathy. Psychiatric symptoms seen in Wilson disease include mood and personality changes, often misinterpreted as puberty-related behavioral changes in children.[56,64,65]

The presence of Kayser-Fleischer (KF) rings is a key diagnostic finding. KF rings are a golden brownish ring formed by the deposition of copper in the Descemet membrane of the cornea.[56] In 98% of cases with neuropsychiatric presentation, KF rings are present.[66] These rings are seen less often in hepatic presentation of this disease, and are usually absent in asymptomatic young individuals.[67] Other rare findings in Wilson disease include arthropathy, hyperparathyroidism, and sunflower cataracts.[68]

Laboratory testing

Serum ceruloplasmin is the screening test most commonly used to evaluate patients suspected of this disease. Values lower than 20 mg/dL along with the presence of KF rings is diagnostic for Wilson disease. The serum ceruloplasmin measurement includes the copper-integrated protein (holoceruloplasmin) and apoceruloplasmin (the precursor to copper incorporation). This protein can be increased by estrogen and is an acute-phase reactant. Thus, the values can be normal in acute liver inflammation and in women taking contraceptive pills.[56] The levels can be falsely low in heterozygotes, patients with rare neurologic diseases, and those with other chronic liver and kidney diseases.[69]

The 24-hour urine copper level is also very helpful. As the free copper (normally 10%) levels increase, the albumin-bound copper is excreted in higher amounts, causing significant cupriuresis. Presence of KF rings along with a urine copper level higher than 100 µg/24 h is diagnostic of Wilson disease. It is useful when the ceruloplasmin level is normal, such as in ALF. Using a cutoff value of 40 µg/24 h makes this test more sensitive[67,70] but less specific, as heterozygotes and patients with cholestatic liver diseases can have cupriuesis in this range.[71] In children, the penicillamine challenge test is still used[72] and can be used along with this cutoff value, thereby improving the specificity of this lower cutoff. This test requires administration of 500 mg penicillamine with repeat dosing 12 hours later to calculate 24-hour copper excretion. A copper-excretion rate of greater than 1600 µg/24 h differentiates Wilson disease from other cholestatic liver diseases.[56] The penicillamine challenge test may not be required in children with mild disease, as the Wilson disease scoring system (see later discussion) may suffice.[67]

In ALF caused by Wilson disease, ceruloplasmin levels can be normal, but serum copper levels and 24-hour urine copper levels are usually elevated. Alkaline phosphatase is very low and a ratio of total bilirubin to alkaline phosphatase of less than 4 and aspartate aminotransferase/alanine aminotransferase ratio of greater than 2.2 are considered to be important diagnostic clues.[73]

Liver biopsy

Liver biopsy is not essential for diagnosis; however, it is useful for staging the disease, calculating the hepatic copper concentration when diagnosis is unclear, or ruling out concomitant liver diseases. A hepatic copper concentration greater than 250 µg/g dry weight is diagnostic while a concentration of greater than 75 µg/g dry weight may help in the diagnosis when other clues are also present. This lower cutoff has higher sensitivity but requires the presence of other typical morphologic and electron-microscopy findings on biopsy to be specific for the diagnosis.[74]

The morphology of the liver on biopsy is variable, and may include steatosis (initially microvesicular), hepatocellular ballooning, and, occasionally, presence of Mallory bodies or even interface hepatitis with prominent plasma cells (as seen in acute on chronic liver failure).[75] Therefore, the diagnosis can be confused with NASH and autoimmune hepatitis.[75,76] Copper staining is performed with the help of dimethylaminobenzylidene rhodanine stain.[77] It may be negative in the earlier stages of disease, when Timm silver stain is more sensitive.[78] The copper in Wilson disease stains in a periseptal pattern and can also stain within nodules, unlike for other cholestatic liver diseases whereby it is only seen in a periportal pattern.[79]

Genetic testing

The discovery of the ATP7B gene has brought about a change in the diagnostic workup of this disease. Liver biopsy is no longer considered necessary for confirmation, and has been replaced by genetic testing in most cases where diagnosis is uncertain. Liver biopsy is still useful for prognostic purposes. ATP7B is the only gene causative for Wilson disease, and more than 95% of patients carry mutations in this gene.[80] The testing is performed by direct sequencing of the 21 exons, which has shown that certain mutations are more prevalent in particular ethnic groups. R778L is seen in Asian populations (Taiwanese, Japanese, and Korean),[81–83] whereas H1069Q is predominantly seen in European Caucasians.[84] Genetic testing is also very useful in identifying affected siblings (who do not have the clinical or biochemical phenotype) of affected patients.[85]

A scoring system incorporating clinical presentation, laboratory testing, histology, and genetic testing was developed 12 years ago at an international conference in Leipzig, Germany.[86] This scoring system provides 1 point each for all the aforementioned diagnostic tests. It has been validated by a recent study that showed that a score of 4 or more is consistent with the diagnosis. This study by Nicastro and colleagues[67] reported a positive and negative predictive value of 93% and 92%, respectively, for this scoring system.

Treatment

The treatment of Wilson disease has improved greatly over the years. It was considered a fatal disease until the observation in 1948 by J.N. Cummings that British antilewisite (BAL) might be useful in the treatment of Wilson disease.[87] In the next 2 decades, D-penicillamine and trientine came onto the market after the pioneering work performed by John Walshe.[88] While D-penicillamine leads to acute cupriuresis, it also induces hepatic metallothionein in the long term, causing mobilization of copper from the liver.[89] Approximately 30% of patients discontinue D-penicillamine because of side effects such as hypersensitivity reactions leading to fever, rash, and proteinuria.[51] It can also cause bone marrow and renal toxicity resulting in aplasia and nephrotic syndrome, respectively. Pyridoxine supplementation is required along with this medication.[90] Trientine has similar efficacy but is much better tolerated, with a significantly lower discontinuation rate and minimal side effects.[91,92] The dosing of both medications is progressively increased until the maximum dose of 20 mg/kg/d is reached. When the patient starts showing improvement in hepatic and neuropsychiatric symptoms, the dose can be decreased by 25% of the maximum dose.[56] Neurologic deterioration has been reported with the use of both of these chelators in patients with predominantly neurologic symptoms.[91] It is not clear whether this is a side effect of these chelators caused by disruption of copper homeostasis, or if it is due to their inability to mobilize copper from the central nervous system.

Zinc salts (sulfate, gluconate, acetate) are occasionally added to these chelators for possible maintenance therapy.[56] Zinc works by inducing metallothionein, which is present in intestinal cells and prevents absorption of dietary copper because of its strong affinity for it.[93] In milder or asymptomatic cases, zinc can also be used as monotherapy.[94] The main disadvantage of zinc therapy is gastrointestinal side effects. Zinc is usually safer in patients with neurologic symptoms, but hepatic decompensation has been reported when it is used as monotherapy, possible because of inefficacious removal of copper.[95]

Ultimately, the goal of treatment is to achieve negative copper balance, which can be followed by periodically checking 24-hour urine copper levels. Once these levels reach 200 to 500 µg/d, the patient can be switched to maintenance therapy (zinc salts or decrease in chelators to maintenance dose). If the 24-hour copper levels are found to be lower than 200 µg/d, overtreatment or noncompliance is possible. Checking serum copper (non–ceruloplasmin-bound copper) helps differentiates this finding. If It is more than 15 µg/dL, patient is likely noncompliant and if it is less than 5 µg/dL, excessive copper is being removed and the dosage of chelator may need to be reduced.[56]

Ammonium tetrathiomolybdate is a noncommercially available compound that combines the action of zinc and the chelators, and the few studies that have evaluated it as a decoppering agent have shown that it has good steady control over free copper levels[96] and has better efficacy than trientine in Wilson disease patients with neurological symptoms.[97,98] Moreover the risk of neurological deterioration is lower than that of other chelators.[96–98] It can lead to few adverse effects such as bone marrow toxicity and elevation in aminotransferases.[99]

Transplant and Survival

Wilson Disease can lead to ALF, which is universally fatal without treatment and almost always entails emergent referral for liver transplant. The post-transplant prognosis is excellent in Wilson disease and it is better in children (1 year survival 90%–100%) and in those with chronic disease (1 year survival 90%–94% in adults).[99] Patients with ALF have better prognosis than those with acute on chronic liver failure.[100] Chelation can lead to reversal of fibrosis and the outcomes with treatment have been evaluated with different prognostic scoring systems.[70,101]

REFERENCES

1. Pietrangelo A, Montosi G, Garuti C, et al. Iron-induced oxidant stress in nonparenchymal liver cells: mitochondrial derangement and fibrosis on acutely iron-dosed gerbils and its prevention by silybin. J Bioenerg Biomembr 2002; 34(1):67–79.
2. Lloyd DR, Philips DH. Oxidative DNA damage mediated by copper(II), iron(II) and nickel(II) fenton reactions: evidence for site-specific mechanisms in the formation of double-strand breaks, 8-hydroxydeoxyguanosine and putative intrastrand cross-links. Mutat Res 1999;424(1–2):23–36.
3. Eaton JW, Qian MW. Molecular bases of cellular iron toxicity. Free Radic Biol Med 2002;32(9):833–40.
4. Gaetke LM, Chow CK. Copper toxicity, oxidative stress, and antioxidant nutrients. Toxicology 2003;189(1–2):147–63.
5. Krumschnabel G, Manzl C, Berger C, et al. Oxidative stress, mitochondrial permeability transition, and cell death in Cu-exposed trout hepatocytes. Toxicol Appl Pharmacol 2005;209(1):62–73.
6. Kono S. Aceruloplasminemia. Curr Drug Targets 2012;13(9):1190–9.
7. Fleming RE, Feng Q, Britton RS. Knockout mouse models of iron homeostasis. Annu Rev Nutr 2011;21(31):117–37.
8. Pietrangelo A. Hereditary hemochromatosis: pathogenesis, diagnosis, and treatment. Gastroenterology 2010;139(2):393–408.
9. Pietrangelo A. Hemochromatosis: an endocrine liver disease. Hepatology 2007; 46(4):1291–301.
10. Nemeth E, Tuttle MS, Powelson J, et al. Hepcidin regulates cellular iron efflux by binding to ferroportin and inducing its internalization. Science 2004;306(5704): 2090–3.
11. Feder JN, Gnirke A, Thomas W, et al. A novel MHC class I-like gene is mutated in patients with hereditary haemochromatosis. Nat Genet 1996;13(4):399–408.
12. Bacon BR, Olynyk JK, Brunt EM, et al. HFE genotype in patients with hemochromatosis and other liver diseases. Ann Intern Med 1999;130(12):953–62.
13. Merryweather-Clarke AT, Pointon JJ, Shearman JD, et al. Global prevalence of putative haemochromatosis mutations. J Med Genet 1997;34(4):275–8.
14. Gochee PA, Powell LW, Cullen DJ, et al. A population-based study of the biochemical and clinical expression of the H63D hemochromatosis mutation. Gastroenterology 2002;122(3):646–51.

15. Cheng R, Barton JC, Morrison ED, et al. Differences in hepatic phenotype between hemochromatosis patients with HFE C282Y homozygosity and other HFE genotypes. J Clin Gastroenterol 2009;43(6):569–73.
16. EASL clinical practice guidelines for HFE hemochromatosis. J Hepatol 2010; 53(1):3–22.
17. Rossi E, Olynyk JK, Jeffrey GP. Clinical penetrance of C282Y homozygous HFE hemochromatosis. Expert Rev Hematol 2008;1(2):205–16.
18. Kowdley KV. Iron, hemochromatosis, and hepatocellular carcinoma. Gastroenterology 2004;127(5 Suppl 1):S79–86.
19. Adams PC, Reboussin DM, Barton JC, et al. Hemochromatosis and iron-overload screening in a racially diverse population. N Engl J Med 2005; 352(17):1769–78.
20. Bassett ML, Halliday JW, Ferris RA, et al. Diagnosis of hemochromatosis in young subjects: predictive accuracy of biochemical screening tests. Gastroenterology 1984;87(3):628–33.
21. Beaton MD, Adams PC. Treatment of hyperferritinemia. Ann Hepatol 2012;11(3): 294–300.
22. Adams PC, McLaren CE, Speechley M, et al. HFE mutations in Caucasian participants of the Hemochromatosis and Iron Overload Screening study with serum ferritin level <1000 μg/L. Can J Gastroenterol 2013;27(7): 390–2.
23. Adams PC, Passmore L, Chakrabarti S, et al. Liver diseases in the hemochromatosis and iron overload screening study. Clin Gastroenterol Hepatol 2006;4(7): 918–23.
24. Allen KJ, Gurrin LC, Constantine CC, et al. Iron-overload-related disease in HFE hereditary hemochromatosis. N Engl J Med 2008;358(3):221–30.
25. Allen KJ, Bertalli NA, Osborne NJ, et al. HFE Cys282Tyr homozygotes with serum ferritin concentrations below 1000 microg/L are at low risk of hemochromatosis. Hepatology 2010;52(3):925–33.
26. Barton JC, Barton JC, Acton RT, et al. Increased risk of death from iron overload among 422 treated probands with HFE hemochromatosis and serum levels of ferritin greater than 1000 μg/L at diagnosis. Clin Gastroenterol Hepatol 2012; 10(4):412–6.
27. Pietrangelo A. Non-HFE hemochromatosis. Hepatology 2004;39:21–9.
28. Pietrangelo A, Caleffi A, Corradini E. Non-HFE hepatic iron overload. Semin Liver Dis 2011;31(3):302–18.
29. Bacon BR, Adams PC, Kowdley KV, et al. Diagnosis and management of hemochromatosis: 2011 practice guideline by the American Association for the Study of Liver Diseases. Hepatology 2011;54(1):328–43.
30. St. Pierre TG, Clarke PR, Chua-Anusorn W. Noninvasive measurement and imaging of liver iron concentrations using proton magnetic resonance. Blood 2005;105(2):855–61.
31. Gandon Y, Olivie D, Guyader D, et al. Non-invasive assessment of hepatic iron stores by MRI. Lancet 2004;363(9406):357–62.
32. Emond MJ, Bronner MP, Carlson TH, et al. Quantitative study of the variability of hepatic iron concentrations. Clin Chem 1999;45(3):340–6.
33. Deugnier Y, Turlin B. Pathology of hepatic iron overload. Semin Liver Dis 2011; 31(3):260–71.
34. Adhoute X, Foucher J, Laharie D, et al. Diagnosis of liver fibrosis using Fibro-Scan and other noninvasive methods in patients with hemochromatosis: a prospective study. Gastroenterol Clin Biol 2008;32(2):180–7.

35. Crawford DH, Murphy TL, Ramm LE, et al. Serum hyaluronic acid with serum ferritin accurately predicts cirrhosis and the need for liver biopsy in C282Y hemochromatosis. Hepatology 2009;49(2):418–25.
36. Bomford A, Williams R. Long term results of venesection therapy in idiopathic hemochromatosis. Q J Med 1976;45(180):611–23.
37. Falize L, Guillygomarc'h A, Perrin M, et al. Reversibility of hepatic fibrosis in treated genetic hemochromatosis: a study of 36 cases. Hepatology 2006;44(2):472–7.
38. Kelly TM, Edwards CQ, Meikle AW, et al. Hypogonadism in hemochromatosis: reversal with iron depletion. Ann Intern Med 1984;101(5):629–32.
39. Cundy T, Butler J, Bomford A, et al. Reversibility of hypogonadotrophic hypogonadism associated with genetic haemochromatosis. Clin Endocrinol (Oxf) 1993; 38(6):617–20.
40. Ko C, Siddaiah N, Berger J, et al. Prevalence of hepatic iron overload and association with hepatocellular cancer in end-stage liver disease: results from the National Hemochromatosis Transplant Registry. Liver Int 2007;27(10):1394–401.
41. Lynch SR, Skikne BS, Cook JD. Food iron absorption in idiopathic hemochromatosis. Blood 1989;74(6):2187–93.
42. Phatak P, Brissot P, Wurster M, et al. A phase 1/2, dose-escalation trial of deferasirox for the treatment of iron overload in HFE-related hereditary hemochromatosis. Hepatology 2010;52(5):1671–9.
43. Rombout-Sestrienkona E, Van Noord PA, Van Deursen CT, et al. Therapeutic erythrocytapheresis versus phlebotomy in the initial treatment of hereditary hemochromatosis—a pilot study. Transfus Apher Sci 2007;36(3):261–7.
44. Bardou-Jacquet E, Philip J, Lorho R, et al. Liver transplantation normalizes serum hepcidin level and cures iron metabolism alterations in HFE hemochromatosis. Hepatology 2013. [Epub ahead of print].
45. Yang Q, McDonnell SM, Khoury MJ, et al. Hemochromatosis-associated mortality in the United States from 1979 to 1992: an analysis of multiple-cause mortality data. Ann Intern Med 1998;129(11):946–53.
46. Niederau C, Fischer R, Sonnenberg A, et al. Survival and causes of death in cirrhotic and in noncirrhotic patients with primary hemochromatosis. N Engl J Med 1985;313(20):1256–62.
47. Milman N, Pedersen P, á Steig T, et al. Clinically overt hereditary hemochromatosis in Denmark 1948-1985: epidemiology, factors of significance for long-term survival, and causes of death in 179 patients. Ann Hematol 2001;80(12):737–44.
48. Phatak PD, Bonkovsky HL, Kowdley KV. Hereditary hemochromatosis: time for targeted screening. Ann Intern Med 2008;149(4):270–2.
49. Adams PC. Implications of genotyping of spouses to limit investigation of children in genetic hemochromatosis. Clin Genet 1998;53(3):176–8.
50. Kanwar P, Kowdley KV. Diagnosis and treatment of hereditary hemochromatosis: an update. Expert Rev Gastroenterol Hepatol 2013;7(6):517–30.
51. European Association for Study of Liver. EASL Clinical Practice Guidelines: Wilson's disease. J Hepatol 2012;56(3):671–85.
52. Coffey AJ, Durkie M, Hague S, et al. A genetic study of Wilson's disease in the United Kingdom. Brain 2013;136(Pt 5):1476–87.
53. Tanzi RE, Petrukhin K, Chernov I, et al. The Wilson disease gene is a copper transporting ATPase with homology to the Menkes disease gene. Nat Genet 1993;5(4):344–50.
54. Yamaguchi Y, Heiny ME, Gitlin JD. Isolation and characterization of a human liver cDNA as a candidate gene for Wilson disease. Biochem Biophys Res Commun 1993;197(1):271–7.

55. Petrukhin K, Fischer SG, Pirastu M, et al. Mapping, cloning and genetic characterization of the region containing the Wilson disease gene. Nat Genet 1993; 5(4):338–43.
56. Roberts EA, Schilsky ML. Diagnosis and treatment of Wilson disease: an update. Hepatology 2008;47(6):2089–111.
57. Wilson SA. Progressive lenticular degeneration: familial nervous disease associated with cirrhosis of liver. Brain 1912;34:295–509.
58. Gowers WR. Tetanoid chorea associated with cirrhosis of liver. Dis Nerv System 1888;2:656.
59. Petrukhin K, Lutsenko S, Chernov I, et al. Characterization of the Wilson disease gene encoding a P-type copper transporting ATPase: genomic organization, alternative splicing, and structure/function predictions. Hum Mol Genet 1994; 3(9):1647–56.
60. Mercer JF. The molecular basis of copper-transport diseases. Trends Mol Med 2001;7(2):64–9.
61. Linder MC, Hazegh-Azam M. Copper biochemistry and molecular biology. Am J Clin Nutr 1996;63(5):797S–811S.
62. Mufti AR, Burstein E, Csomos RA, et al. XIAP Is a copper binding protein deregulated in Wilson's disease and other copper toxicosis disorders. Mol Cell 2006;21(6):775–85.
63. Dabrowska E, Jabłońska-Kaszewska I, Ozieblowski A, et al. Acute haemolytic syndrome and liver failure as the first manifestations of Wilson's disease. Med Sci Monit 2001;7(Suppl 1):246–51.
64. Rosencrantz R, Schilsky M. Wilson disease: pathogenesis and clinical considerations in diagnosis and treatment. Semin Liver Dis 2011;31(3):245–59.
65. Huster D. Wilson disease. Best Pract Res Clin Gastroenterol 2010;24(5):531–9.
66. Steindl P, Ferenci P, Dienes HP, et al. Wilson's disease in patients presenting with liver disease: a diagnostic challenge. Gastroenterology 1997;113(1):212–8.
67. Nicastro E, Ranucci G, Vajro P, et al. Re-evaluation of the diagnostic criteria for Wilson disease in children with mild liver disease. Hepatology 2010;52(6): 1948–56.
68. Ferenci P. Pathophysiology and clinical features of Wilson disease. Metab Brain Dis 2004;19(3–4):229–39.
69. Walshe JM. Diagnostic significance of reduced serum caeruloplasmin concentration in neurological disease. Mov Disord 2005;20(12):1658–61.
70. Dhawan A, Taylor RM, Cheeseman P, et al. Wilson's disease in children: 37-year experience and revised King's score for liver transplantation. Liver Transpl 2005; 11(4):441–8.
71. Frommer DJ. Urinary copper excretion and hepatic copper concentrations in liver disease. Digestion 1981;21(4):169–78.
72. Martins da Costa C, Baldwin D, et al. Value of urinary copper excretion after penicillamine challenge in the diagnosis of Wilson's disease. Hepatology 1992;15(4): 609–15.
73. Korman JD, Volenberg I, Balko J, et al, Pediatric and Adult Acute Liver Failure Study Groups. Screening for Wilson disease in acute liver failure: a comparison of currently available diagnostic tests. Hepatology 2008;48(4):1167–74.
74. Ferenci P, Steindl-Munda P, Vogel W, et al. Diagnostic value of quantitative hepatic copper determination in patients with Wilson's disease. Clin Gastroenterol Hepatol 2005;3(8):811–8.
75. Johncilla M, Mitchell KA. Pathology of the liver in copper overload. Semin Liver Dis 2011;31(3):239–44.

76. Milkiewicz P, Saksena S, Hubscher SG, et al. Wilson's disease with superimposed autoimmune features: report of two cases and review. J Gastroenterol Hepatol 2000;15(5):570–4.
77. Irons RD, Schenk EA, Lee JC. Cytochemical methods for copper. Semiquantitative screening procedure for identification of abnormal copper levels in liver. Arch Pathol Lab Med 1977;101(6):298–301.
78. Pilloni L, Lecca S, Van Eyken P, et al. Value of histochemical stains for copper in the diagnosis of Wilson's disease. Histopathology 1998;33(1):28–33.
79. Salaspuro MP, Pikkarainen P, Sipponen P, et al. Hepatic copper in primary biliary cirrhosis: biliary excretion and response to penicillamine treatment. Gut 1981; 22(11):901–6.
80. Bennett J, Hahn SH. Clinical molecular diagnosis of Wilson disease. Semin Liver Dis 2011;31(3):233–8.
81. Chuang LM, Wu HP, Jang MH, et al. High frequency of two mutations in codon 778 in exon 8 of the ATP7B gene in Taiwanese families with Wilson disease. J Med Genet 1996;33(6):521–3.
82. Nanji MS, Nguyen VT, Kawasoe JH, et al. Haplotype and mutation analysis in Japanese patients with Wilson disease. Am J Hum Genet 1997;60(6):1423–9.
83. Kim EK, Yoo OJ, Song KY, et al. Identification of three novel mutations and a high frequency of the Arg778Leu mutation in Korean patients with Wilson disease. Hum Mutat 1998;11(4):275–8.
84. Thomas GR, Forbes JR, Roberts EA, et al. The Wilson disease gene: spectrum of mutations and their consequences. Nat Genet 1995;9(2):210–7.
85. Manolaki N, Nikolopoulou G, Daikos GL, et al. Wilson disease in children: analysis of 57 cases. J Pediatr Gastroenterol Nutr 2009;48(1):72–7.
86. Ferenci P, Caca K, Loudianos G, et al. Diagnosis and phenotypic classification of Wilson disease. Liver Int 2003;23(3):139 42.
87. Cumings JN. The effects of B.A.L. in hepatolenticular degeneration. Brain 1951; 74(1):10–22.
88. Purchase R. The treatment of Wilson's disease, a rare genetic disorder of copper metabolism. Sci Prog 2013;96(Pt 1):19–32.
89. Scheinberg IH, Sternlieb I, Schilsky M, et al. Penicillamine may detoxify copper in Wilson's disease. Lancet 1987;2(8550):95.
90. Aaseth J, Flaten TP, Andersen O. Hereditary iron and copper deposition: diagnostics, pathogenesis and therapeutics. Scand J Gastroenterol 2007;42(6):673–81.
91. Weiss KH, Thurik F, Gotthardt DN, et al. Efficacy and safety of oral chelators in treatment of patients with Wilson disease. Clin Gastroenterol Hepatol 2013; 11(8):1028–35.
92. Taylor RM, Chen Y, Dhawan A, et al. Triethylene tetramine dihydrochloride (trientine) in children with Wilson disease: experience at King's College Hospital and review of the literature. Eur J Pediatr 2009;168(9):1061–8.
93. Hall AC, Young BW, Bremner I. Intestinal metallothionein and the mutual antagonism between copper and zinc in the rat. J Inorg Biochem 1979;11(1):57–66.
94. Czlonkowska A, Gajda J, Rodo M. Effects of long-term treatment in Wilson's disease with D-penicillamine and zinc sulphate. J Neurol 1996;243(3):269–73.
95. Weiss KH, Gotthardt DN, Klemm D, et al. Zinc monotherapy is not as effective as chelating agents in treatment of Wilson disease. Gastroenterology 2011;140(4): 1189–98.
96. Brewer GJ, Askari F, Dick RB, et al. Treatment of Wilson's disease with tetrathiomolybdate: V. Control of free copper by tetrathiomolybdate and a comparison with trientine. Transl Res 2009;154(2):70–7.

97. Brewer GJ, Hedera P, Kluin KJ, et al. Treatment of Wilson disease with ammonium tetrathiomolybdate: III. Initial therapy in a total of 55 neurologically affected patients and follow-up with zinc therapy. Arch Neurol 2003;60(3):379–85.

98. Brewer GJ, Askari F, Lorincz MT, et al. Treatment of Wilson disease with ammonium tetrathiomolybdate: IV. Comparison of tetrathiomolybdate and trientine in a double-blind study of treatment of the neurologic presentation of Wilson disease. Arch Neurol 2006;63(4):521–7.

99. Arnon R, Annunziato R, Schilsky M, et al. Liver transplantation for children with Wilson disease: comparison of outcomes between children and adults. Clin Transplant 2011;25(1):E52–60.

100. Thanapirom K, Treeprasertsuk S, Komolmit P, et al. Comparison of long-term outcome of patients with Wilson's disease presenting with acute liver failure versus acute-on-chronic liver failure. J Med Assoc Thai 2013;96(2):150–6.

101. Nazer H, Ede RJ, Mowat AP, et al. Wilson's disease: clinical presentation and use of prognostic index. Gut 1986;27(11):1377–81.

Hepatocellular Carcinoma and Other Liver Lesions

Reena Salgia, MD[a], Amit G. Singal, MD, MS[b,c],*

KEYWORDS

- Liver cancer • Liver mass • Diagnosis • Treatment

KEY POINTS

- Hepatocellular carcinoma (HCC) is the most common primary liver tumor, with most cases developing in a background of cirrhosis or chronic hepatitis B virus infection.
- Benign liver lesions and other malignancies, such as cholangiocarcinoma, should be considered in the differential diagnosis of a liver mass, particularly in patients without pre-existing chronic liver disease.
- The most common modality for diagnosis of HCC is contrast-enhanced magnetic resonance imaging or 4-phase computed tomography, with characteristic findings of arterial enhancement and delayed phase washout.
- The Barcelona Clinic Liver Cancer staging system is endorsed by the American Association for the Study of Liver Diseases and remains the most commonly used staging system in clinical practice.
- Treatment decisions for HCC should be individualized after accounting for a patient's tumor burden, liver function, and performance status. Given the multitude of potential treatment options, a multidisciplinary approach to care is recommended for optimal communication and treatment delivery.

INTRODUCTION

Hepatocellular carcinoma (HCC) is currently the sixth most prevalent cancer worldwide and the third leading cause of cancer-related death.[1] It is one of the leading causes of morbidity and mortality in patients with cirrhosis. Furthermore, it has a rapidly rising incidence in the United States and Europe, largely driven by the burden of advanced hepatitis C virus (HCV) and nonalcoholic steatohepatitis (NASH) cases.[2,3]

Disclosures: Dr Singal is on the speaker bureau for Bayer/Onyx Pharmaceuticals.
[a] Division of Gastroenterology and Hepatology, Henry Ford Hospital, 2799 West Grand Boulevard, Suite K7, Detroit, MI 48202, USA; [b] Division of Digestive and Liver Diseases, University of Texas Southwestern Medical Center, 5959 Harry Hines Boulevard, POB 1, Suite 420, Dallas, TX, USA; [c] Harold C Simmons Cancer Center, University of Texas Southwestern Medical Center, 2201 Inwood Road, Dallas, TX 75390, USA
* Corresponding author. Division of Digestive and Liver Diseases, University of Texas Southwestern Medical Center, 5959 Harry Hines Boulevard, POB 1, Suite 420, Dallas, TX 75390-8887.
E-mail address: amit.singal@utsouthwestern.edu

Med Clin N Am 98 (2014) 103–118
http://dx.doi.org/10.1016/j.mcna.2013.09.003
0025-7125/14/$ – see front matter © 2014 Elsevier Inc. All rights reserved.

Prognosis for patients with HCC depends on tumor stage at diagnosis, with curative options available only for patients diagnosed at an early stage. Unfortunately, two-thirds of patients with HCC are diagnosed at an advanced stage, when curative options no longer exist and median survival is less than 1 year.[4,5] Despite improvements in therapy, prognosis for patients with HCC remains poor, with 5-year survival rates of only 18%.[4,6] With increasing availability of new treatment options for patients with HCC, treatment decisions have become more complex and challenging.[7] The aim of this review was to provide an up-to-date summary of the diagnosis and management of HCC.

RISK FACTORS

More than 90% of HCC develop in patients with chronic liver disease.[3,8,9] Cirrhosis, the most well-recognized risk factor, is associated with an annual risk of 2% to 7%.[10] HCV-associated cirrhosis is the causative agent largely responsible for the increase in incidence of HCC in the United States and Europe. The incidence of HCC in patients with HCV cirrhosis is up to 2% to 6% per year, although this can be significantly decreased by successful antiviral therapy.[11,12] However, the most frequent risk factor for HCC worldwide is chronic HBV infection, accounting for more than 50% of all cases.[13] Other risk factors include older age, male gender, obesity, diabetes, aflatoxin exposure, and alcohol and tobacco use.[14,15] However, predictive models for HCC based on these known risk factors have been limited by modest accuracy to date, and further refinement is still needed before their routine use in clinical practice.[11,16–18] Inclusion of novel biomarkers or genetic risk factors might improve HCC risk stratification.

SURVEILLANCE

Surveillance for HCC is recommended in high-risk populations, most notably patients with cirrhosis. The goal of surveillance is to detect tumors at an early stage when they are amenable to curative therapy so as to reduce mortality.[8,19] A randomized controlled trial (RCT) from China demonstrated a survival benefit with surveillance using ultrasound and alpha fetoprotein (AFP) in patients with chronic hepatitis B virus infection.[20] Although a similar RCT has not been performed in patients with cirrhosis, several prospective cohort studies, after adjusting for lead-time bias, have demonstrated that cirrhotic patients undergoing surveillance have earlier stages of disease and better survival than patients who had not undergone surveillance.[21–23] However, fewer than 20% of patients with cirrhosis undergo HCC surveillance, contributing to high rates of advanced tumor stage at presentation.[24–26]

The American Association for the Study of Liver Disease (AASLD) endorses HCC surveillance in high-risk patients using ultrasound alone every 6 months.[8] Although ultrasound has a pooled sensitivity of 63% for detecting HCC at an early stage in prospective cohort studies, its sensitivity in clinical practice is substantially lower at 32%.[27–29] AFP appears to be beneficial in clinical practice, increasing sensitivity for early-stage HCC to 63.4%, when used in combination with ultrasound.[28] Although investigators are attempting to identify novel biomarkers, a large multicenter study demonstrated that AFP, at a cutoff of 10.9 ng/mL, is more sensitive for early-stage HCC than other biomarkers, including des-gamma carboxy-prothrombin (DCP) and lens culinaris-agglutinin reactive fraction of AFP (AFP-L3).[30] Further studies are needed to better evaluate the potential role of new biomarkers before their routine use in clinical practice. Until that time, ultrasound and AFP remain the optimal HCC surveillance strategy.

DIAGNOSIS AND STAGING

Fig. 1 shows the diagnostic algorithm for patients with suspected HCC.[8] Lesions smaller than 1 cm in diameter can be challenging to confidently diagnose. Given the potential harm of liver biopsy and low risk of HCC, close observation with a repeat ultrasound in 3 months is sufficient.[31,32] If a nodule larger than1 cm is detected, further evaluation should be performed using contrast-enhanced magnetic resonance imaging (MRI) or 4-phase computed tomography (CT).

The typical imaging pattern for HCC on CT or MRI is a hypervascular lesion during the arterial phase, followed by hypointensity (or contrast washout) during the portal venous and delayed phase. If the appearance of a lesion is typical for HCC, this is sufficient for diagnosis and no further investigation is necessary. If the appearance is not typical for HCC, a second contrast-enhanced study or biopsy should be performed to establish the diagnosis. Patients with a high suspicion for HCC but a negative biopsy should continue to be followed with serial contrast-enhanced imaging. If the lesion enlarges but remains atypical appearing, a repeat biopsy should be considered. In one study validating this approach, the false-negative rate was as high as 30% and up to 3 biopsies were required in some cases to confirm the diagnosis.[33]

Cancer staging is critical to provide patients with prognostic information and to determine the appropriate management strategy. Although there is not one universally

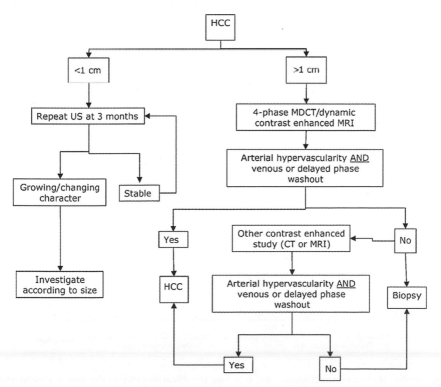

Fig. 1. Diagnostic algorithm for hepatocellular carcinoma. MDCT, multidetector computed tomography; US, ultrasound. (*From* Bruix J, Sherman M. Management of hepatocellular carcinoma: an update. Hepatology 2010;53:8; with permission.)

accepted staging system, the Barcelona Clinic Liver Cancer (BCLC) staging system is the most accepted in clinical practice because it includes an assessment of tumor burden, liver function, and performance status.[8,34] The BCLC is also unique, as it is the only staging system linking tumor stage with an evidence-based treatment algorithm (**Fig. 2**).

SYMPTOMS

The clinical presentation of HCC varies widely and is largely driven by the degree of underlying hepatic reserve. In patients with cirrhosis, HCC can present with hepatic decompensation, including hepatic encephalopathy, ascites, or jaundice.[35] In patients with adequate hepatic reserve and particularly those without cirrhosis, HCC is more likely to present with tumor-related symptoms, including abdominal pain, weight loss, weakness, anorexia, malaise, or a palpable mass on examination. Of these potential symptoms, a dull visceral abdominal pain is the most common symptom. Whereas small tumors are often asymptomatic, HCC typically becomes symptomatic when it reaches 5 to 8 cm in diameter.[22,36] Because nearly 40% of patients can have HCC as their first presentation of cirrhosis, identification of chronic liver disease and cirrhosis before the development of HCC is of paramount importance.[37]

Extrahepatic manifestations of HCC can result from distant metastases or a paraneoplastic syndrome. The most common sites of extrahepatic metastases include lung, abdominal lymph nodes, and bone.[38,39] Paraneoplastic syndromes are rare in early HCC but are reported in up to 40% of patients with large tumors and high AFP levels. Potential paraneoplastic phenomena include hypoglycemia, erythrocytosis, hypercalcemia, hypercholesterolemia, and thrombocytopenia.[40]

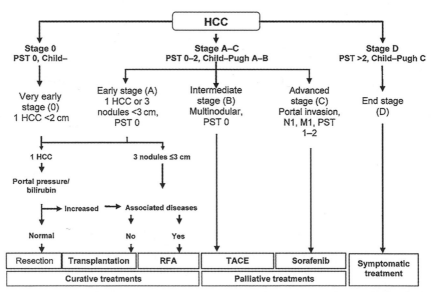

Fig. 2. Treatment algorithm for patients with HCC using the Barcelona Clinic Liver Cancer Staging System. M, metastasis classification; N, node classification; PST, performance status; RFA, radiofrequency ablation; TACE, transarterial chemoembolization. (*From* Bruix J, Sherman M. Management of hepatocellular carcinoma: an update. Hepatology 2010;53:14; with permission.)

DIFFERENTIAL DIAGNOSIS

There are other malignant and benign liver lesions that can present in patients with or without cirrhosis (**Table 1**).

Malignant Lesions

The most common cause of multiple liver masses is metastasis from a nonhepatic primary malignancy. These may be solitary, multiple, or occasionally even infiltrative lesions. The most common tumor to metastasize to the liver is colorectal adenocarcinoma. Other tumors that commonly metastasize to the liver include renal cell carcinoma, melanoma, breast cancer, thyroid cancer, lung cancer, gastroesophageal tumors, and neuroendocrine tumors. The appearance of metastases on imaging can be varied, either hypovascular or hypervascular depending on the etiology of the primary tumor. Multiphase MRI with T1-weighted and T2-weighted images is the preferred diagnostic modality.

Intrahepatic cholangiocarcinoma is the second most common primary liver tumor. Resection remains the most effective option for long-term disease-free survival, although only 19% to 74% are resectable due to advanced tumor burden at the time of diagnosis.[41] For highly selected patients with localized hilar cholangiocarcinoma, liver transplantation may also be an option.[42] Posttransplant survival has improved over time, with 5-year survival rates approaching 59% after 2000.[43] For patients in whom resection or transplantation are not options, chemoradiation is the mainstay of management. However, data regarding chemoradiotherapy do not demonstrate a clear benefit, as survival is rarely extended beyond the projected 6 to 15 months.[44]

Fibrolamellar HCC is a rare variant of HCC. Patients are typically young (<30 years old) and often do not have underlying liver disease. Fibrolamellar HCC is slower growing than conventional HCC and often presents with pain or a palpable mass once the lesion is large. On imaging, fibrolamellar HCC tends to be nonencapsulated or well circumscribed. For localized disease, prognosis tends to be better than conventional HCC, with high rates of resectability.

Benign Lesions

Hemangioma is the most common benign liver lesion. It is most often diagnosed in the fourth to sixth decades of life and has a female predominance. It can be solitary or multifocal and is often diagnosed incidentally on imaging performed for other reasons. Giant variants can occupy an entire hepatic lobe and on rare occasion can hemorrhage. Contrast-enhanced imaging shows peripheral arterial enhancement with

Table 1 Differential diagnosis of liver lesions	
Benign	**Malignant**
Hepatic cysts[a]	Hepatocellular carcinoma
Biliary hamartoma	Fibrolamellar hepatocellular carcinoma
Pyogenic abscess	Nonhepatic metastatic disease
Nonpyogenic abscess	Intrahepatic cholangiocarcinoma
Hemangioma	
Hepatic adenoma[b]	
Focal nodular hyperplasia	

[a] With the exception of mucinous cystadenomas.
[b] Rare malignant potential reported.

central filling on venous and delayed images.[45] Diagnosis is usually made by the characteristic imaging features, and biopsy is not recommended because of their highly vascular nature. Intervention is needed only if patients are symptomatic, in which case surgical resection is recommended. These lesions do not have malignant potential and no routine follow-up is required.

Focal nodular hyperplasia (FNH) is another benign liver lesion with female predominance and no malignant potential. They represent a hyperplastic response of the liver parenchyma, with a disorganized growth of hepatocytes and bile ducts. Contrast-enhanced imaging shows an intense homogeneous enhancement in the arterial phase, followed by isointense venous phase and enhancement of the central scar in later phases.[45] These are usually diagnosed incidentally on imaging, and follow-up is rarely required. In rare cases, patients may become symptomatic, in which case resection can be considered with excellent outcomes.[46]

Hepatic adenomas are benign liver lesions, with female predominance and mean age of diagnosis in the fourth decade. They are often solitary lesions, but can be found in multiples. Risk factors for development and growth include use of oral contraceptives, pregnancy, anabolic steroid use, and glycogen storage diseases. Contrast-enhanced imaging shows a well-demarcated lesion that is lipid-rich, often containing glycogen. There is early hyperintensity, with delayed images showing an isointense or hypointense lesion. Areas of prior hemorrhage, necrosis, or calcifications may be present.[45] Hepatic adenomas typically remain stable in size and patients remain asymptomatic. However, discontinuation of oral contraceptives and/or steroid use is strongly recommended, with serial monitoring by imaging. Risk of intralesional hemorrhage or rupture can be as high as 26%, and is most common in lesions 5 cm or larger, exophytic lesions, subcapsular position, or those with prior evidence of hemorrhage.[47] There is also the low but reported risk of 4% for malignant transformation, particularly for lesions larger than 5 cm.[48] Surgical resection can be considered for symptomatic lesions, lesions larger than 5 cm in diameter, and those increasing in size despite the discontinuation of oral contraceptives and steroids.[49] Other management options include bland embolization, ablation, and, in rare cases, liver transplantation. There are promising pathomolecular markers, which may allow for better identification of high-risk lesions that require resection in the future.[50,51]

Hepatic cysts are commonly found in adults and can be congenital or acquired. Most commonly these are simple cysts, but other variants include polycystic liver diseases, hemorrhagic cysts, parasitic cysts, biliary hamartomas, and rarely cystic neoplasms. On MRI, simple cysts have high T2 signal with a uniform smooth border and lack of enhancement on postcontrast images.[52] Cysts may occasionally contain septations, lobulation, or contain debris owing to protein or posthemorrhage contents. Biliary hamartomas are benign, usually peripherally located in the liver, composed of small irregular branching bile ducts in a fibrous stroma, and may have peripheral rim enhancement on MRI. In contrast to cystic neoplasms or solid metastatic lesions, these lesions do not have progressive internal enhancement.[53] Cystic neoplasms, such as a mucinous cystadenocarcinoma, often show distinctive postcontrast enhancement around the rim of the lesion with variable central enhancement on delayed images.[45]

Hepatic abscesses can develop from several infectious agents, although a detailed discussion of these lesions is beyond the scope of this review. The most important include pyogenic abscesses and nonpyogenic abscesses (amebic, echinococcal, mycobacterial, or fungal). Pyogenic abscesses contain central purulent necrosis with a rind of granulation tissue. Most commonly these arise from bacterial organisms entering the portal venous system from a bowel source and seeding the liver.[54] The most common cause of infectious granuloma worldwide is tuberculosis, although various mycobacterial organisms can invade the liver. Amebic abscesses due to *Entamoeba histolytica* are rare in industrialized countries and usually are acquired during travel to endemic or tropical areas. Echinococcal abscesses can result from 2 organisms, which form a hydatid cyst. Imaging reveals a large parent cyst with daughter cysts. If the cyst ruptures and fluid leaks, a significant inflammatory reaction can develop.[55] Finally, fungal organisms, such as *Candida* species, can form liver abscesses but are generally limited to immunocompromised patients.

MANAGEMENT AND TREATMENT
Early-stage HCC

Patients with early-stage HCC have the most favorable prognosis, given the availability of curative options. Surgical resection is the treatment of choice for patients with HCC but no history of cirrhosis. However, most patients with HCC in the United States have underlying cirrhosis, so widespread use of resection is limited. Patients with cirrhosis are at risk for hepatic decompensation following resection if they do not have adequate hepatic reserve, so careful patient selection is crucial. It is important to consider both quality and quantity of the future liver remnant (FLR) after resection. In patients with limited fibrosis, the risk of postoperative morbidity is low if FLR exceeds 30%; however, an FLR of 40% is typically required in patients with cirrhosis.[56] If the size of the FLR is a concern, portal vein embolization can be performed to promote hypertrophy of the unaffected lobe.[57] Quality of FLR is based on an assessment of hepatic function and degree of portal hypertension. Survival at 5 years is reported to be 74% after resection in patients without portal hypertension or hyperbilirubinemia, compared with 25% for patients with these conditions.[58]

Although resection has been associated with 5-year survival rates of nearly 70%, the risk of recurrence is as high as 50% at 5 years.[59] In the early period (ie, within 2 years of resection), recurrence is most likely related to dissemination from the original tumor; late recurrences (ie, those occurring more than 2 years after resection) likely represent "de novo" HCC, particularly when in a background of cirrhosis.[60,61] Use of neoadjuvant therapy, including transarterial chemoembolization (TACE), does not prolong survival in cases of resectable HCC, and could increase dropout rates due to interval disease progression.[62]

Liver transplantation is the only therapeutic option for HCC that treats both the tumor and corrects the underlying cirrhosis. Priority listing is designated for patients in the United States who meet "Milan criteria" (ie, 1 tumor smaller than 5 cm in size or 2 to 3 tumors, each smaller than 3 cm without vascular invasion or extrahepatic spread). When these criteria are applied, the recurrence rate of HCC is typically less than 15% and 5-year survival rates are near 68%.[63] Patients with T2 HCC who are listed for transplantation are eligible for additional model for end-stage liver disease points to gain priority on the waiting list. Locoregional therapy is often used as a bridge while patients are awaiting transplantation to reduce the risk of dropout, particularly in regions with long wait times, although there is no proven posttransplant survival benefit.[64,65]

Some believe the Milan criteria may be too restrictive and have proposed expanding selection criteria to include patients with larger tumors. The University of California San Francisco (UCSF) criteria includes patients with a single lesion smaller than 6.5 cm or 2 to 3 lesions, each smaller than 4.5 cm with a maximum tumor burden of 8.0 cm.[66] The "up-to-7" criteria include patients whose sum of the largest tumor diameter and number of tumors is less than 7.[67] However, the benefit of considering patients who exceed Milan criteria must be weighed against the harm of delaying transplantation in other patients on the waiting list.[68] Patients who exceed Milan criteria have higher posttransplant mortality (hazard ratio [HR] 1.68, 95% confidence interval [CI] 1.39–2.03) than those within Milan criteria, with 5-year posttransplant survival rates of only 38%.[69] Alternatively, patients with large tumors can be considered for "downstaging" to fit within Milan criteria by using percutaneous ablation, TACE, or transarterial radioembolization (TARE). A prospective study of 61 patients with locally advanced tumors who exceeded transplant criteria (1 lesion >5 cm and ≤8 cm, 2–3 lesions with 1 lesion >3 cm but ≤5 cm and total tumor volume ≤8 cm, or 4–5 lesions with all ≤3 cm and total tumor volume ≤8 cm) showed that downstaging was successful in approximately 70% of patients.[70] The 4-year survival of the entire cohort was 69% and 92% in the 35 patients who underwent transplantation.

For patients with early HCC who do not qualify for resection or transplantation, the best option is percutaneous local ablative therapy. Radiofrequency ablation (RFA) has become the most frequently used form of local ablative therapy. RFA achieves higher rates of complete tumor ablation than percutaneous ethanol injection (PEI) using fewer sessions, with tumor necrosis rates of 90% to 95% in solitary HCCs smaller 4 cm.[71–75] A meta-analysis also demonstrated that 3-year survival is significantly prolonged with RFA compared with PEI (odds ratio [OR] 0.48, 95% CI 0.34–0.67).[76]

Three RCTs demonstrated similar 3-year survival rates between percutaneous ablation and resection in patients with early HCC, although there was a consistent trend in higher disease-free survival after resection.[77–79] Local expertise should be considered when deciding between these 2 options. A Markov model using these data concluded that resection is the best therapeutic option except if patients are older than 70 years, peri-operative mortality for resection exceeds 30%, negative margins are achieved less than 60% of the time, or if RFA can be performed in most recurrence cases.[80]

Intermediate-stage HCC

TACE is the standard treatment for patients with intermediate-stage HCC. The liver derives most of its blood flow from the portal vein, whereas HCCs are dependent on hepatic artery blood supply. Taking advantage of this difference in blood supply, TACE involves selective delivery of intra-arterial chemotherapy into the tumor, followed by embolization with a goal of inducing tissue necrosis. TACE results in a significantly prolonged 2-year survival of 63% compared with 27% with supportive care (P<.001).[81] A postembolization syndrome due to local tissue ischemia occurs in up to 50% of patients with fevers, nausea, and abdominal pain as the predominant symptoms.[82] There is high variability in procedural technique, including choice of chemotherapeutic agent (doxorubicin alone vs combination with mitomycin-C or 5-fluorouracil vs bland embolization), embolizing agent (gel foam vs microparticles), TACE re-treatment schedule (ranging from every 2 months–6 months), and degree of selectivity (ranging from super-selective to lobar TACE). The introduction of drug-eluting beads (DEB-TACE), which can be more embolic and maintain higher intratumor doxorubicin levels, may reduce some of the heterogeneity between sites. An RCT among 212 patients with intermediate-stage HCC found DEB-TACE had similar response rates to conventional TACE (27% vs 22% complete response) and similar treatment-related serious adverse effects rates.[83] A recent study of 104 patients treated with DEB-TACE validated the safety (9.6% major complication rate) and efficacy (median survival 48.6 months) of DEB-TACE.[84]

TARE using yttrium-90 microspheres has been introduced to target radiation therapy to the tumor while limiting exposure to the nontumor parenchyma. During TARE, radiolabeled particles are injected through the hepatic artery and become trapped at the precapillary level and emit internal radiation. In a single-center prospective

Table 2
Phase II clinical trials for patients with advanced HCC[a]

Drug Regimen	Mechanism of Action
First-line therapy (treatment-naïve patients)	
Capecitabine and oxaliplatin[b]	Antineoplastic, inhibits DNA synthesis
S-1 and leucovorin	Antineoplastic, inhibits DNA synthesis
Tegafururacil[b]	Antineoplastic, inhibits DNA synthesis
Doxorubicin[b]	Antineoplastic, intercalates DNA to prevent replication
TH-302[b]	Antineoplastic, hypoxia activated radical anion prodrug
OPB-31121	Antineoplastic, inhibits STAT3 phosphorylation
mFOLFOX[b]	Antineoplastic
TS-1 and oxaliplatin	Antineoplastic
Temsirolimus[b]	mTOR inhibitor
Temsirolimus and bevacizumab	mTOR inhibitor (temsirolimus) Angiogenesis inhibitor (bevacizumab)
Everolimus and SOM230	mTOR inhibitor (everolimus) Somatostatin analog (SOM230)
Axitinib	Multityrosine kinase inhibitor
Dasatinib	Multityrosine kinase inhibitor
E7050[b]	Dual kinase inhibitor
PD 0332991	Cyclin-dependent kinase Inhibitor
INC280	cMET-receptor tyrosine kinase inhibitor
BIBF 1120	Angiokinase inhibitor
Tivozanib	Tyrosine kinase inhibitor
Erlotinib and bevacizumab	Tyrosine kinase inhibitor (erlotinib) Angiogenesis inhibitor (bevacizumab)
Bavituximab[b]	Monoclonal antibody targeting phospholipids
R05137382 (GC33)	Recombinant monoclonal antibody against glypican-3
VT-122[b]	Beta-blocker plus COX2 selective enzyme inhibitor
SOM230 (pasireotide)	Somatostatin analog
Pravastatin[b]	HMG-CoA reductase inhibitor
G-202	Cytoxin directed at tumor vasculature
Second-line therapy (patients who fail sorafenib)	
MK2206	Antineoplastic – allosteric AKT inhibitor
ABT-888 and temozolomide	Antineoplastic, inhibits Poly ADP ribose polymerase (ABT-888) Oral ankylating agent (temozolomide)
SGI-110	Antineoplastic, inhibits DNA synthesis
Lenalidomide	Antineoplastic, induces tumor cell apoptosis, antiangiogenic, and antiosteoclastogenic
Temsirolimus	mTOR inhibitor
TRC105[b]	Anti endoglin monoclonal antibody
TRC105	Anti-endoglin monoclonal antibody

Abbreviations: COX, cyclo-oxygenase; mTOR, mammalian target of rapamycin.
[a] From http://www.clinicaltrials.gov; includes studies with status verified within the past 12 months and/or actively recruiting patients.
[b] Used in combination with sorafenib.

study of 291 patients treated with TARE, 23% had complete response and 34% partial response.[85] Median survival in this cohort was 17.2 months for Child Pugh A patients and 7.7 months for Child Pugh B patients. In a follow-up study comparing TARE (n = 123) and TACE (n = 122), there was no significant difference in tumor response rates (49% vs 36%, P = .10) or median survival (20.5 vs 17.4 months, P = .23).[86]

Advanced-stage HCC

To date, sorafenib is the only systemic therapy shown to prolong survival in patients with advanced-stage HCC. In 2008, the SHARP trial was the first RCT to demonstrate a significant survival benefit in these patients.[87] Median survival was shown to improve from 7.9 months with placebo to 10.7 months with sorafenib. Most patients in this trial had Child Pugh A cirrhosis (95%) and good performance status (92%) with advanced tumors (53% extrahepatic spread and 70% vascular invasion). Overall, sorafenib appears well tolerated, with the most common adverse effects including diarrhea, hand-foot skin reaction, and anorexia/weight loss. A postmarketing study assessing tolerability and outcomes with sorafenib in clinical practice revealed Child Pugh B patients experienced a higher rate of serious adverse events than Child Pugh A patients (60% vs 33%) but similar incidence of drug-related serious adverse events (16% vs 10%).[88] However, patients with Child Pugh C cirrhosis or poor performance status are unlikely to tolerate the therapy or derive significant benefit.[89] Trials are ongoing to determine any benefit of adding sorafenib to other treatment modalities, such as surgical resection or TACE, and/or for the treatment of posttransplant HCC recurrence.

There have been several trials evaluating other targeted therapies for advanced HCC. Other targeted therapies that were previously studied but failed in phase III trials include sunitinib,[90] which did not demonstrate superiority or noninferiority to sorafenib, and brivanib, which failed to demonstrate improved survival compared with placebo.[91,92] Although promising results have been seen for other agents in phase II studies, none have been confirmed to date in large phase III studies (**Table 2**). Although patient cohorts in most of these studies are small and unselected, research into molecularly targeted therapy is rapidly expanding.

Multidisciplinary Management

Treatment decisions for HCC have become increasingly complex with the availability of novel therapies and the growing use of multimodal and multiprovider treatments. Appropriate treatment decisions, individualized for each patient, require the complementary expertise of multiple specialties. A multidisciplinary approach involving a team of hepatologists, surgeons, interventional radiologists, radiation oncologists, medical oncologists, and radiologists can improve communication and allow delivery of optimal treatment.

SUMMARY AND FUTURE CONSIDERATIONS

Cirrhosis is the most well recognized risk factor for HCC and is present in more than 90% of HCC cases in the United States. Unfortunately, patients with HCC are often diagnosed at an advanced stage, emphasizing the importance of surveillance in high-risk patients to identify HCC at earlier stages of disease. Contrast-enhanced MRI or 4-phase CT is recommended for evaluation of any suspicious liver lesions. The BCLC is most commonly used staging system in clinical practice to determine HCC stage and management options. There have been many advances in treatment options for HCC over the past few years, including increased uptake of TARE and development of molecular targeted therapies. In the future, we are likely to see further investigation into the value of adjuvant and neoadjuvant therapies with resection or transplantation, as well as development of novel targeted systemic therapies. There are now possible therapies for most patients with any stage of disease; however, treatment decisions must be individualized after accounting for factors such as degree of liver dysfunction and patient performance status. Treatment decisions for HCC are likely to remain complex and require an ongoing multidisciplinary approach to care.

REFERENCES

1. Ferlay J, Shin HR, Bray F, et al. Estimates of worldwide burden of cancer in 2008: GLOBOCAN 2008. Int J Cancer 2010;127:2893–917.
2. El-Serag HB. Epidemiology of viral hepatitis and hepatocellular carcinoma. Gastroenterology 2012;142:1264–73.e1.
3. El-Serag HB, Rudolph KL. Hepatocellular carcinoma: epidemiology and molecular carcinogenesis. Gastroenterology 2007;132:2557–76.
4. Altekruse SF, McGlynn KA, Reichman ME. Hepatocellular carcinoma incidence, mortality, and survival trends in the United States from 1975 to 2005. J Clin Oncol 2009;27:1485–91.
5. Llovet JM, Bustamante J, Castells A, et al. Natural history of untreated nonsurgical hepatocellular carcinoma: rationale for the design and evaluation of therapeutic trials. Hepatology 1999;29:62–7.
6. Altekruse SF, McGlynn KA, Dickie LA, et al. Hepatocellular carcinoma confirmation, treatment, and survival in surveillance, epidemiology, and end results registries, 1992-2008. Hepatology 2012;55:476–82.
7. Padhya KT, Marrero JA, Singal AG. Recent advances in the treatment of hepatocellular carcinoma. Curr Opin Gastroenterol 2013;29:285–92.
8. Bruix J, Sherman M. Management of hepatocellular carcinoma: an update. Hepatology 2010;53:1–35.
9. Yang JD, Kim WR, Coelho R, et al. Cirrhosis is present in most patients with hepatitis B and hepatocellular carcinoma. Clin Gastroenterol Hepatol 2011;9:64–70.
10. Collier J, Sherman M. Screening for hepatocellular carcinoma. Hepatology 1998;27:273–8.
11. Lok AS, Seeff LB, Morgan TR, et al. Incidence of hepatocellular carcinoma and associated risk factors in hepatitis C-related advanced liver disease. Gastroenterology 2009;136:138–48.
12. Singal AG, Volk ML, Jensen D, et al. A sustained viral response is associated with reduced liver-related morbidity and mortality in patients with hepatitis C virus. Clin Gastroenterol Hepatol 2010;8:280–8, 288.e1.
13. Beasley R. Hepatitis B virus. The major etiology of hepatocellular carcinoma. Cancer 1988;61:1942–56.
14. El-Serag HB, Tran T, Everhart JE. Diabetes increases the risk of chronic liver disease and hepatocellular carcinoma. Gastroenterology 2004;126:460–8.
15. Marrero JA, Fontana RJ, Fu S, et al. Alcohol, tobacco and obesity are synergistic risk factors for hepatocellular carcinoma. J Hepatol 2005;42:218–24.
16. Lee E, Edward S, Singal AG, et al. Improving screening for hepatocellular carcinoma by incorporating data on levels of alpha-fetoprotein, over time. Clin Gastroenterol Hepatol 2013;11:437–40.
17. Singal AG, Waljee A, Mukherjee A, et al. Machine learning algorithms outperform conventional regression models in identifying risk factors for hepatocellular carcinoma in patients with cirrhosis. Gastroenterology 2012;142:S984.

18. Velazquez RF, Rodriguez M, Navascues CA, et al. Prospective analysis of risk factors for hepatocellular carcinoma in patients with liver cirrhosis. Hepatology 2003;37:520–7.
19. Bruix J, Sherman M, Llovet JM, et al. Clinical management of hepatocellular carcinoma. Conclusions of the Barcelona-2000 EASL conference. European Association for the Study of the Liver. J Hepatol 2001;35:421–30.
20. Zhang BH, Yang BH, Tang ZY. Randomized controlled trial of screening for hepatocellular carcinoma. J Cancer Res Clin Oncol 2004;130:417–22.
21. El-Serag HB, Kramer JR, Chen GJ, et al. Effectiveness of AFP and ultrasound tests on hepatocellular carcinoma mortality in HCV-infected patients in the USA. Gut 2011;60:992–7.
22. Trevisani F, De NS, Rapaccini G, et al. Semiannual and annual surveillance of cirrhotic patients for hepatocellular carcinoma: effects on cancer stage and patient survival (Italian experience). Am J Gastroenterol 2002;97: 734–44.
23. Wong GL, Wong VW, Tan GM, et al. Surveillance programme for hepatocellular carcinoma improves the survival of patients with chronic viral hepatitis. Liver Int 2008;28:79–87.
24. Davila JA, Henderson L, Kramer JR, et al. Utilization of surveillance for hepatocellular carcinoma among hepatitis C virus-infected veterans in the United States. Ann Intern Med 2011;154:85–93.
25. Davila JA, Morgan RO, Richardson PA, et al. Use of surveillance for hepatocellular carcinoma among patients with cirrhosis in the United States. Hepatology 2010;52:132–41.
26. Singal AG, Yopp A, S Skinner C, et al. Utilization of hepatocellular carcinoma surveillance among American patients: a systematic review. J Gen Intern Med 2012;27:861–7.
27. Singal A, Volk ML, Waljee A, et al. Meta-analysis: surveillance with ultrasound for early-stage hepatocellular carcinoma in patients with cirrhosis. Aliment Pharmacol Ther 2009;30:37–47.
28. Singal AG, Conjeevaram HS, Volk ML, et al. Effectiveness of hepatocellular carcinoma surveillance in patients with cirrhosis. Cancer Epidemiol Biomarkers Prev 2012;21:793–9.
29. Singal AG, Nehra M, Adams-Huet B, et al. Detection of hepatocellular carcinoma at advanced stages among patients in the HALT-C trial: where did surveillance fail? Am J Gastroenterol 2013;108:425–32.
30. Marrero JA, Feng Z, Wang Y, et al. Alpha-fetoprotein, des-gamma carboxyprothrombin, and lectin-bound alpha-fetoprotein in early hepatocellular carcinoma. Gastroenterology 2009;137:110–8.
31. Iwasaki M, Furuse J, Yoshino M, et al. Sonographic appearances of small hepatic nodules without tumor stain on contrast-enhanced computed tomography and angiography. J Clin Ultrasound 1998;26:303–7.
32. Jeong YY, Mitchell DG, Kamishima T. Small (<20 mm) enhancing hepatic nodules seen on arterial phase MR imaging of the cirrhotic liver: clinical implications. AJR Am J Roentgenol 2002;178:1327–34.
33. Forner A, Vilana R, Ayuso C, et al. Diagnosis of hepatic nodules 20 mm or smaller in cirrhosis: prospective validation of the noninvasive diagnostic criteria for hepatocellular carcinoma. Hepatology 2008;47:97–104.
34. Marrero JA, Fontana RJ, Barrat A, et al. Prognosis of hepatocellular carcinoma: comparison of 7 staging systems in an American cohort. Hepatology 2005;41: 707–16.

35. Trevisani F, D'Intino PE, Caraceni P, et al. Etiologic factors and clinical presentation of hepatocellular carcinoma. Differences between cirrhotic and noncirrhotic Italian patients. Cancer 1995;75:2220–32.
36. Yuen MF, Cheng CC, Lauder IJ, et al. Early detection of hepatocellular carcinoma increases the chance of treatment: Hong Kong experience. Hepatology 2000;31:330–5.
37. Singal AG, Yopp AC, Gupta S, et al. Failure rates in the hepatocellular carcinoma surveillance process. Cancer Prev Res (Phila) 2012;5:1124–30.
38. Katyal S, Oliver JH 3rd, Peterson MS, et al. Extrahepatic metastases of hepatocellular carcinoma. Radiology 2000;216:698–703.
39. Lee YT, Geer DA. Primary liver cancer: pattern of metastasis. J Surg Oncol 1987; 36:26–31.
40. Luo JC, Hwang SJ, Wu JC, et al. Clinical characteristics and prognosis of hepatocellular carcinoma patients with paraneoplastic syndromes. Hepatogastroenterology 2002;49:1315–9.
41. Singal AG, Rakoski MO, Salgia R, et al. The clinical presentation and prognostic factors for intrahepatic and extrahepatic cholangiocarcinoma in a tertiary care centre. Aliment Pharmacol Ther 2010;31:625–33.
42. Darwish Murad S, Kim WR, Harnois DM, et al. Efficacy of neoadjuvant chemoradiation, followed by liver transplantation, for perihilar cholangiocarcinoma at 12 US centers. Gastroenterology 2012;143:88–98.e3 [quiz: e14].
43. Salgia RJ, Singal AG, Fu S, et al. Improved post-transplant survival in the United States for patients with cholangiocarcinoma after 2000. Dig Dis Sci 2013. [Epub ahead of print].
44. Glimelius B, Hoffman K, Sjoden PO, et al. Chemotherapy improves survival and quality of life in advanced pancreatic and biliary cancer. Ann Oncol 1996;7: 593–600.
45. Bilgili Y, Firat Z, Pamuklar E, et al. Focal liver lesions evaluated by MR imaging. Diagn Interv Radiol 2006;12:129–35.
46. Hsee LC, McCall JL, Koea JB. Focal nodular hyperplasia: what are the indications for resection? HPB (Oxford) 2005;7:298–302.
47. van Aalten SM, de Man RA, IJzermans JN, et al. Systematic review of haemorrhage and rupture of hepatocellular adenomas. Br J Surg 2012;99:911–6.
48. Stoot JH, Coelen RJ, De Jong MC, et al. Malignant transformation of hepatocellular adenomas into hepatocellular carcinomas: a systematic review including more than 1600 adenoma cases. HPB (Oxford) 2010;12:509–22.
49. Ault GT, Wren SM, Ralls PW, et al. Selective management of hepatic adenomas. Am Surg 1996;62:825–9.
50. Bioulac-Sage P, Balabaud C, Zucman-Rossi J. Subtype classification of hepatocellular adenoma. Dig Surg 2010;27:39–45.
51. Nault JC, Bioulac-Sage P, Zucman-Rossi J. Hepatocellular benign tumors—from molecular classification to personalized clinical care. Gastroenterology 2013; 144:888–902.
52. Martin DR, Semelka RC. Imaging of benign and malignant focal liver lesions. Magn Reson Imaging Clin N Am 2001;9:785–802, vi–vii.
53. Semelka RC, Hussain SM, Marcos HB, et al. Biliary hamartomas: solitary and multiple lesions shown on current MR techniques including gadolinium enhancement. J Magn Reson Imaging 1999;10:196–201.
54. Heneghan HM, Healy NA, Martin ST, et al. Modern management of pyogenic hepatic abscess: a case series and review of the literature. BMC Res Notes 2011; 4:80.

55. Karavias D, Panagopoulos C, Vagianos C, et al. Infected echinococcal cyst. A common cause of pyogenic hepatic abscess. Ups J Med Sci 1988;93:289–96.
56. Farges O, Malassagne B, Flejou JF, et al. Risk of major liver resection in patients with underlying chronic liver disease: a reappraisal. Ann Surg 1999;229:210–5.
57. de Graaf W, van Lienden KP, van den Esschert JW, et al. Increase in future remnant liver function after preoperative portal vein embolization. Br J Surg 2011;98:825–34.
58. Llovet JM, Fuster J, Bruix J. Intention-to-treat analysis of surgical treatment for early hepatocellular carcinoma: resection versus transplantation. Hepatology 1999;30:1434–40.
59. Poon RT. Optimal initial treatment for early hepatocellular carcinoma in patients with preserved liver function: transplantation or resection? Ann Surg Oncol 2007;14:541–7.
60. Poon RT, Fan ST, Ng IO, et al. Different risk factors and prognosis for early and late intrahepatic recurrence after resection of hepatocellular carcinoma. Cancer 2000;89:500–7.
61. Portolani N, Coniglio A, Ghidoni S, et al. Early and late recurrence after liver resection for hepatocellular carcinoma: prognostic and therapeutic implications. Ann Surg 2006;243:229–35.
62. Zhou WP, Lai EC, Li AJ, et al. A prospective, randomized, controlled trial of pre-operative transarterial chemoembolization for resectable large hepatocellular carcinoma. Ann Surg 2009;249:195–202.
63. Onaca N, Davis GL, Jennings LW, et al. Improved results of transplantation for hepatocellular carcinoma: a report from the International Registry of Hepatic Tumors in Liver Transplantation. Liver Transpl 2009;15:574–80.
64. Lesurtel M, Mullhaupt B, Pestalozzi BC, et al. Transarterial chemoembolization as a bridge to liver transplantation for hepatocellular carcinoma: an evidence-based analysis. Am J Transplant 2006;6:2644–50.
65. Thuluvath PJ, Guidinger MK, Fung JJ, et al. Liver transplantation in the United States, 1999-2008. Am J Transplant 2010;10:1003–19.
66. Yao FY, Ferrell L, Bass NM, et al. Liver transplantation for hepatocellular carcinoma: expansion of the tumor size limits does not adversely impact survival. Hepatology 2001;33:1394–403.
67. Mazzaferro V, Llovet JM, Miceli R, et al. Predicting survival after liver transplantation in patients with hepatocellular carcinoma beyond the Milan criteria: a retrospective, exploratory analysis. Lancet Oncol 2009;10:35–43.
68. Volk ML, Vijan S, Marrero JA. A novel model measuring the harm of transplanting hepatocellular carcinoma exceeding Milan criteria. Am J Transplant 2008;8:839–46.
69. Mazzaferro V, Bhoori S, Sposito C, et al. Milan criteria in liver transplantation for hepatocellular carcinoma: an evidence-based analysis of 15 years of experience. Liver Transpl 2011;17(Suppl 2):S44–57.
70. Yao FY, Kerlan RK Jr, Hirose R, et al. Excellent outcome following down-staging of hepatocellular carcinoma prior to liver transplantation: an intention-to-treat analysis. Hepatology 2008;48:819–27.
71. Brunello F, Veltri A, Carucci P, et al. Radiofrequency ablation versus ethanol injection for early hepatocellular carcinoma: a randomized controlled trial. Scand J Gastroenterol 2008;43:727–35.
72. Lin SM, Lin CJ, Lin CC, et al. Radiofrequency ablation improves prognosis compared with ethanol injection for hepatocellular carcinoma < or = 4 cm. Gastroenterology 2004;127:1714–23.

73. Lin SM, Lin CJ, Lin CC, et al. Randomised controlled trial comparing percutaneous radiofrequency thermal ablation, percutaneous ethanol injection, and percutaneous acetic acid injection to treat hepatocellular carcinoma of 3 cm or less. Gut 2005;54:1151–6.
74. Livraghi T, Goldberg SN, Lazzaroni S, et al. Hepatocellular carcinoma: radiofrequency ablation of medium and large lesions. Radiology 2000;214:761–8.
75. Shiina S, Teratani T, Obi S, et al. A randomized controlled trial of radiofrequency ablation with ethanol injection for small hepatocellular carcinoma. Gastroenterology 2005;129:122–30.
76. Cho YK, Kim JK, Kim MY, et al. Systematic review of randomized trials for hepatocellular carcinoma treated with percutaneous ablation therapies. Hepatology 2009;49:453–9.
77. Chen MS, Li JQ, Zheng Y, et al. A prospective randomized trial comparing percutaneous local ablative therapy and partial hepatectomy for small hepatocellular carcinoma. Ann Surg 2006;243:321–8.
78. Huang GT, Lee PH, Tsang YM, et al. Percutaneous ethanol injection versus surgical resection for the treatment of small hepatocellular carcinoma: a prospective study. Ann Surg 2005;242:36–42.
79. Lu MD, Kuang M, Liang LJ, et al. Surgical resection versus percutaneous thermal ablation for early-stage hepatocellular carcinoma: a randomized clinical trial. Zhonghua Yi Xue Za Zhi 2006;86:801–5.
80. Molinari M, Helton S. Hepatic resection versus radiofrequency ablation for hepatocellular carcinoma in cirrhotic individuals not candidates for liver transplantation: a Markov model decision analysis. Am J Surg 2009;198:396–406.
81. Llovet JM, Real MI, Montana X, et al. Arterial embolisation or chemoembolisation versus symptomatic treatment in patients with unresectable hepatocellular carcinoma: a randomised controlled trial. Lancet 2002;359:1734–9.
82. Pomoni M, Malagari K, Moschouris H, et al. Post embolization syndrome in doxorubicin eluting chemoembolization with DC bead. Hepatogastroenterology 2012;59:820–5.
83. Lammer J, Malagari K, Vogl T, et al. Prospective randomized study of doxorubicin-eluting-bead embolization in the treatment of hepatocellular carcinoma: results of the PRECISION V study. Cardiovasc Intervent Radiol 2010; 33:41–52.
84. Burrel M, Reig M, Forner A, et al. Survival of patients with hepatocellular carcinoma treated by transarterial chemoembolisation (TACE) using drug eluting Beads. Implications for clinical practice and trial design. J Hepatol 2012;56: 1330–5.
85. Salem R, Lewandowski RJ, Mulcahy MF, et al. Radioembolization for hepatocellular carcinoma using yttrium-90 microspheres: a comprehensive report of long-term outcomes. Gastroenterology 2010;138:52–64.
86. Salem R, Lewandowski RJ, Kulik L, et al. Radioembolization results in longer time-to-progression and reduced toxicity compared with chemoembolization in patients with hepatocellular carcinoma. Gastroenterology 2011;140: 497–507.e2.
87. Llovet JM, Ricci S, Mazzaferro V, et al. Sorafenib in advanced hepatocellular carcinoma. N Engl J Med 2008;359:378 90.
88. Lencioni R, Kudo M, Ye SL, et al. First interim analysis of the GIDEON (Global Investigation of therapeutic decisions in hepatocellular carcinoma and of its treatment with sorafenib) non-interventional study. Int J Clin Pract 2012;66: 675–83.

89. Worns MA, Weinmann A, Pfingst K, et al. Safety and efficacy of sorafenib in patients with advanced hepatocellular carcinoma in consideration of concomitant stage of liver cirrhosis. J Clin Gastroenterol 2009;43:489–95.

90. Cheng A, Kang YK, Lin D, et al. Phase III trial of sunitinib (Su) versus sorafenib (So) in advanced hepatocellular carcinoma (HCC). J Clin Oncol 2011;29S [abstract 4000].

91. Finn RS, Kang YK, Mulcahy M, et al. Phase II, open-label study of brivanib as second-line therapy in patients with advanced hepatocellular carcinoma. Clin Cancer Res 2012;18:2090–8.

92. Park JW, Finn RS, Kim JS, et al. Phase II, open-label study of brivanib as first-line therapy in patients with advanced hepatocellular carcinoma. Clin Cancer Res 2011;17:1973–83.

Management of End-stage Liver Disease

Iris W. Liou, MD

KEYWORDS

- Cirrhosis - Ascites - Peritonitis - Varices - Hepatic encephalopathy
- Decompensation

KEY POINTS

- Patients with cirrhosis should be referred to a liver transplant center if they (1) have a model for end-stage liver disease score greater than or equal to 10 or Child-Turcotte-Pugh score greater than or equal to 7, (2) develop a complication caused by cirrhosis (eg, ascites, variceal hemorrhage, or hepatic encephalopathy), or (3) are diagnosed with hepatocellular carcinoma within Milan criteria (solitary lesion less than 5 cm or up to 3 nodules each smaller than 3 cm).
- Treatment of ascites in patients with cirrhosis should be focused on dietary sodium restriction of less than 2000 mg daily and the use of diuretics; specifically, spironolactone and furosemide, titrated using a respective ratio of 100 mg to 40 mg.
- An ascitic fluid absolute polymorphonuclear (PMN) count greater than or equal to 250 cells/mm^3 should prompt empiric antibiotic treatment of spontaneous bacterial peritonitis with intravenous cefotaxime (2 g intravenously every 8 hours) for 5 days.
- Nonselective β-blockers (NSBBs) are recommended for the prevention of the first variceal hemorrhage in those with large esophageal varices or small esophageal varices at high risk of bleeding (red wale marks or Child class B or C cirrhosis). Endoscopic variceal ligation can be performed for large esophageal varices when NSBBs are contraindicated or not tolerated.
- Lactulose can be used as initial drug therapy for the treatment of acute hepatic encephalopathy, even in the absence of high-quality, placebo-controlled trials, based on extensive clinical experience supporting efficacy. Rifaximin is a reasonable alternative in those who do not respond to lactulose alone.
- Patients with cirrhosis should undergo ultrasound imaging every 6 months for hepatocellular carcinoma surveillance.

INTRODUCTION

Cirrhosis is a progressive, diffuse fibrotic process in the liver, leading to nodule formation and disruption of the normal architecture, and can result from any chronic insult to

No financial disclosures.
Division of Gastroenterology, Department of Medicine, University of Washington School of Medicine, 1959 Northeast Pacific Street, Box 356175, Seattle, WA 98195-6175, USA
E-mail address: irisl@medicine.washington.edu

Med Clin N Am 98 (2014) 119–152
http://dx.doi.org/10.1016/j.mcna.2013.09.006
0025-7125/14/$ – see front matter
© 2014 Elsevier Inc. All rights reserved.

the liver. Specific liver diseases that can lead to cirrhosis include chronic viral hepatitis (eg, hepatitis B and hepatitis C), autoimmune hepatitis, alcoholic liver disease, cholestatic liver diseases (eg, primary biliary cirrhosis, primary sclerosing cholangitis, and cystic fibrosis), metabolic disorders (eg, alpha-1-antitrypsin deficiency, Wilson disease, nonalcoholic steatohepatitis, and hereditary hemochromatosis), and vascular disorders (eg, Budd-Chiari syndrome). Well-compensated cirrhosis can remain asymptomatic for many years until a decompensating event occurs, such as the development of jaundice, ascites, spontaneous bacterial peritonitis, variceal hemorrhage, or hepatic encephalopathy (HE). Once a complication of cirrhosis develops, the 5-year survival decreases to less than 20%, and patients should be referred for consideration of liver transplantation.[1] Liver-related mortality is the 12th leading cause of mortality in the United States, as reported by the National Center for Health Statistics, and, because of under-reporting, the true mortality is likely even higher.[2] The vigilant care of patients with cirrhosis centers on the prevention and management of these events.

ASCITES
Evaluation of Ascites

Ascites is the most common complication of cirrhosis, with approximately 50% of patients with compensated cirrhosis developing ascites over the course of 10 years.[1,3] After the development of ascites necessitating hospitalization, the risk of mortality increases to 15% at 1 year and nearly 50% at 5 years.[4]

History and physical examination
In the United States, approximately 85% of patients with ascites have cirrhosis as the cause of ascites.[5] In addition to the assessment of risk factors for liver disease, a history or risk factors for malignancy, heart failure, nephrotic syndrome, thyroid myxedema, recent abdominal surgery, and tuberculosis should be elicited. Physical examination findings for ascites include bulging flanks and shifting dullness.

Diagnostic and therapeutic paracentesis
The evaluation for the cause of clinically apparent ascites should begin with an abdominal paracentesis with appropriate ascitic fluid analysis. Prophylactic blood products do not routinely need to be given before a paracentesis in patients with cirrhosis with associated thrombocytopenia and coagulopathy.[6,7] The paracentesis procedure is generally safe, with only a 1% risk of abdominal wall hematoma and a less than 0.5% risk of mortality, even in patients with coagulopathy related to liver disease. However, this procedure should be avoided in the setting of clinically evident hyperfibrinolysis or disseminated intravascular coagulation.

Initial evaluation of cause of ascites
The following includes a summary of major laboratory tests to consider performing with diagnostic paracentesis (**Table 1**). Other tests not discussed can be ordered if there is suspicion for alternative or additional causes of ascites.

Albumin and total protein Ascitic fluid sample should routinely be sent for albumin and total protein. The serum-ascites albumin gradient (SAAG) is calculated by subtracting the ascitic fluid albumin value from the serum albumin concentration obtained on the same day. A SAAG value greater than or equal to 1.1 g/dL indicates portal hypertension,[5] but does not exclude additional causes of ascites in a patient with portal hypertension. An ascitic fluid total protein value less than 2.5 g/dL is consistent with ascites from cirrhosis or nephrotic syndrome, whereas a high ascitic fluid protein value greater than 2.5 g/dL is seen in patients with cardiac or thyroid causes of ascites.

Table 1
Differential diagnosis for ascites

Indication	Serum-Ascites Albumin Gradient		Additional Diagnostic Tests
	High (≥1.1 g/dL)	Low (<1.1 g/dL)	
Liver Related			
Cirrhosis	X	—	Ascitic fluid cell count and differential for spontaneous bacterial peritonitis, total protein
Alcoholic hepatitis	X	—	—
Acute liver failure	X	—	—
Budd-Chiari syndrome, hepatic vein occlusion	X	—	Imaging
Sinusoidal obstruction syndrome	X	—	—
Sarcoidosis, hepatic granulomas	X	—	Liver biopsy
Polycystic liver disease	X	—	Imaging
Nodular regenerative hyperplasia	X	—	Liver biopsy
Cardiac (congestive heart failure, constrictive pericarditis, pulmonary hypertension)	X	—	Echocardiogram, right heart catheterization
Neoplasm			
Hepatocellular carcinoma	X	—	Imaging
Liver metastases	X	—	Imaging
Peritoneal carcinomatosis	—	X	Imaging, cytology
Malignant chylous ascites	—	X	Ascitic fluid triglyceride, imaging
Meigs syndrome (benign ovarian tumor)	—	X	Imaging
Infection			
Tuberculous peritonitis	—	X	Directed peritoneal biopsy and mycobacterial culture, ascitic fluid mycobacterial culture
Chlamydia peritonitis	—	X	Imaging, nucleic acid test for chlamydia
Secondary bacterial peritonitis	—	X	Ascitic fluid glucose, LDH, Gram stain, carcinoembryonic antigen, alkaline phosphatase
Nephrotic syndrome	—	X	24-h urine protein
Protein-losing enteropathy	—	X	24-h stool alpha-1-antitrypsin
Pancreatic ascites	—	X	Ascitic fluid amylase
Thyroid myxedema	X	—	Serum thyroid tests
Postoperative lymphatic leak	—	X	Ascitic fluid triglyceride
Biliary peritonitis	—	X	Ascitic fluid bilirubin
Serositis	—	X	—
Bowel obstruction or infarction	—	X	Imaging

Abbreviation: LDH, lactate dehydrogenase.

Data from Runyon BA, Montano AA, Akriviadis EA, et al. The serum-ascites albumin gradient is superior to the exudate-transudate concept in the differential diagnosis of ascites. Ann Intern Med 1992;117:215–20.

Cell count and cultures A cell count and differential should routinely be performed on ascitic fluid. In the case of a traumatic paracentesis, with the entry of blood into the ascitic fluid (typically ascitic red cells greater than 10,000 cells/mm^3), the polymorphonuclear leukocyte (PMN) count should be corrected by subtracting 1 PMN for every 250 red cells/mm^3 from the absolute PMN count. With any concern for infection, the fluid should be directly inoculated into aerobic and anaerobic blood culture bottles at the bedside before the administration of antibiotics, which increases the yield of bacterial growth in culture from 50% to around 80% when the PMN count is greater than or equal to 250 cells/mm^3.[8,9]

Other tests Ascitic fluid carcinoembryonic antigen (CEA), alkaline phosphatase, total protein, glucose, and lactate dehydrogenase (LDH) tests are useful in the diagnosis of secondary bacterial peritonitis.[10] Ascitic fluid cytology is expensive and is only revealing in the setting of peritoneal carcinomatosis. Serum cancer antigen 125 can be increased in any patient with ascites or pleural effusion of any cause, because the level increases when mesothelial cells are under pressure in the presence of fluid, so it does not indicate ovarian malignancy in this setting; thus, it is not helpful as a diagnostic test for ascites.[11]

Persistent ascites caused by cirrhosis Patients undergoing serial outpatient therapeutic paracenteses only need to have the fluid routinely sent for cell count and differential.[12]

Basic Management of Ascites

Sodium restriction and diuretics are the mainstay of treatment of patients with ascites caused by portal hypertension. Patients with low SAAG (less than 1.1 g/dL) ascites do not respond well to these measures, with the exception of those with nephrotic syndrome (**Box 1**).

Treatment of the underlying disorder

Cessation of alcohol use is vital to the management of ascites caused by alcoholic liver disease.[13] Treatment of autoimmune hepatitis and chronic hepatitis B also leads to significant clinical improvement and resolution of ascites in some cases.

Dietary sodium restriction

Patients with portal hypertension–associated ascites should restrict their daily dietary sodium intakes to less than 2000 mg (88 mmol).[14] Any further restriction risks malnutrition caused by poor palatability of foods.

Box 1
Management of ascites caused by cirrhosis

1. Treatment of underlying disorder (eg, alcoholic liver disease, hepatitis B, autoimmune hepatitis)

2. Dietary sodium restriction (less than 2000 mg per day)

3. Diuretic therapy (maintain ratio spironolactone 100 mg to furosemide 40 mg)

4. Therapeutic paracentesis

5. Fluid restriction only if serum sodium less than120 mEq/L or symptomatic hyponatremia

Data from Runyon BA, AASLD. Introduction to the revised American Association for the Study of Liver Diseases Practice Guideline management of adult patients with ascites due to cirrhosis 2012. Hepatology 2013;57:1651–3.

Fluid restriction

Dietary sodium restriction is more important than fluid restriction in the management of cirrhosis. Fluid restriction is not necessary unless the serum sodium concentration is less than 120 mmol/L, or if mental status changes that develop are attributed to hyponatremia.

Diuretics

In patients with portal hypertension, the combination of spironolactone and furosemide, starting at doses of 100 mg daily and 40 mg daily, respectively, is recommended.[15–17] If weight loss is insufficient, the doses of the diuretics may be increased simultaneously every 3 to 5 days, maintaining the 100 mg to 40 mg ratio, to maximum daily doses of 400 mg of spironolactone and 160 mg of furosemide. For patients unable to tolerate spironolactone because of painful gynecomastia, amiloride (10–60 mg daily) can be substituted, although it is less effective.[18] In patients with significant peripheral edema, there is no limit for daily weight loss, but, in those without peripheral edema, weight loss should be restricted to a maximum of 0.5 kg a day.[19]

Medications to be avoided

Because of the lack of efficacy and safety data, vasopressin receptor antagonists are not recommended for the management of ascites.[20] The use of angiotensin-converting enzyme inhibitors and angiotensin receptor blockers should be avoided in patients with cirrhosis, because of concerns of renal failure and increased mortality for those who develop hypotension. In patients with refractory ascites, propranolol is associated with decreased survival, perhaps because of the increased risk of paracentesis-induced circulatory dysfunction, so the risks and benefits of its use should be considered individually for each patient.[21,22] Nonsteroidal antiinflammatory drugs (NSAIDs), including aspirin, should also be avoided because of the risk of reduced urinary sodium excretion and renal failure.

Management of tense ascites

A single large-volume paracentesis followed by dietary sodium restriction and initiation of diuretics is appropriate as initial therapy for new-onset large-volume ascites.[23] Up to 5 L can be removed without significant disturbances in systemic and renal hemodynamics. If more than 5 L of ascitic fluid are removed, then intravenous albumin (8 g per liter of fluid removed) should be given.[24,25]

Management of Refractory Ascites

Less than 20% of patients with cirrhosis and ascites develop refractory ascites.[26] Refractory ascites is defined as ascites that is unresponsive to dietary sodium restriction and maximal diuretic dosing (typically, spironolactone 400 mg daily and furosemide 160 mg daily), or that recurs rapidly after therapeutic paracentesis. Once refractory ascites develops, 1-year mortality is approximately 50%.[27–29]

Serial large-volume therapeutic paracenteses

Once a patient is deemed diuretic resistant, diuretics should be discontinued, and management may rely on serial large-volume therapeutic paracenteses alone.[23] A large-volume paracentesis of up to 10 L removed every 2 weeks typically controls ascites in a patient who is compliant with dietary sodium restriction. Need for more frequent paracenteses suggests dietary noncompliance. Long-term serial paracenteses can lead to significant loss of protein and can worsen malnutrition, but placement of a percutaneous endoscopic gastrostomy tube in an effort to provide nutrition should be avoided in these patients because of the high risk of mortality associated with performing the procedure.[30]

Albumin infusions with therapeutic paracentesis

A meta-analysis of 17 trials showed a reduction in risk of postparacentesis circulatory dysfunction, hyponatremia, and mortality in the albumin group (odds ratio of death 0.64, 95% confidence interval, 0.41–0.98) compared with the nonalbumin group. The studies typically used a protocol of administering 5 to 10 g of albumin per liter of fluid removed, using 20% or higher concentration of albumin solution.[31] Thus, the 6 to 8 g of intravenous albumin per liter of ascitic fluid removed during or immediately following large-volume paracentesis (greater than 5 L removed) should be considered.

Transjugular intrahepatic portosystemic shunt

Transjugular intrahepatic portosystemic shunt (TIPS), a side-to-side portocaval shunt placed intravenously by interventional radiology, has been shown in multiple multicenter randomized controlled trials to be superior to serial large-volume paracenteses in the control of ascites, but with varying results on the impact on overall transplant-free survival and the potential risk of inducing or worsening HE.[32–36] Polytetrafluoroethylene-covered stents are preferred rather than uncovered stents because of decreased rates of TIPS occlusion.

Contraindications The absolute and relative contraindications to placement of TIPS are listed in **Boxes 2** and **3**.[37]

Outcome after TIPS Short-term and long-term mortality following TIPS can be estimated using model for end-stage liver disease (MELD) and Child-Turcotte-Pugh scoring systems, although most of the patients in these studies had TIPS placed for management of variceal bleeding rather than refractory ascites, for which prognosis is expected to be worse. Clinical improvement following TIPS is seen in 75% of patients.[38] Diuretics may need to be continued even after placement of TIPS. Approximately 30% of patients develop HE after TIPS, and most of them can be managed medically (eg, lactulose).

Peritoneovenous shunts

The use of peritoneovenous shunts for management of ascites has fallen out of favor because of limited long-term patency (less than 20% at 2 years), risk of complications, and lack of improvement in survival compared with medical therapy.[26,28] It is reserved as palliative treatment in select patients who are not candidates for transplantation, TIPS, or serial therapeutic paracenteses.

Box 2
Absolute contraindications for TIPS

Congestive heart failure (especially right sided)

Severe tricuspid regurgitation

Severe pulmonary hypertension (mean pulmonary artery pressure greater than 45 mm Hg)

Extensive polycystic liver disease

Uncontrolled infection

Unrelieved biliary obstruction

Data from Boyer TD, Haskal ZJ; American Association for the Study of Liver Diseases. The role of Transjugular Intrahepatic Portosystemic Shunt (TIPS) in the Management of Portal Hypertension: update 2009. Hepatology 2010;51:306.

Box 3
Relative contraindications for TIPS

Complete hepatic vein obstruction

Complete portal vein thrombosis

Hepatocellular carcinoma (especially if centrally located)

Severe coagulopathy (international normalized ratio [INR] greater than 5)

Severe thrombocytopenia (platelet count less than 20,000/cm^3)

Recurrent or severe spontaneous HE

Advanced liver dysfunction (bilirubin greater than 5 mg/dL or model for end-stage liver disease [MELD] greater than 17)

Moderate pulmonary hypertension

Cardiac systolic dysfunction (ejection fraction less than 60%)

Cardiac diastolic dysfunction

Advanced age (greater than 69 years)

Data from Boyer TD, Haskal ZJ, American Association for the Study of Liver Diseases. The role of Transjugular Intrahepatic Portosystemic Shunt (TIPS) in the Management of Portal Hypertension: update 2009. Hepatology 2010;51:306.

Complications Associated with Ascites

Complications following the development of ascites include spontaneous bacterial peritonitis, dilutional hyponatremia, refractory ascites, and hepatorenal syndrome. Development of these complications negatively affects the likelihood of survival.

Spontaneous Bacterial Peritonitis

Spontaneous bacterial peritonitis (SBP) occurs in up to 30% of patients with cirrhosis and ascites, and has an estimated in-hospital mortality of 20%.[39] The prevalence of SBP in cirrhotic outpatients is 1.5% to 3.5% and in inpatients is about 10%.[40] Most cases of SBP are caused by gram-negative enteric organisms, such as *Escherichia coli* and *Klebsiella pneumoniae*.[41]

Indications for testing

In a patient with ascites, new-onset fever (temperature greater than 37.8°C or 100°F), abdominal pain, HE, metabolic acidosis, renal failure, hypotension, diarrhea, paralytic ileus, hypothermia, leukocytosis, or other sign or symptom of infection should prompt a diagnostic paracentesis for ascitic fluid analysis and culture (**Table 2**).[42] Because SBP is so commonly present at the time of any type of admission for a cirrhotic patient, a diagnostic paracentesis is recommended routinely for these patients at the time of admission.[43]

Diagnostic criteria

The diagnosis of confirmed SBP requires an increased ascitic fluid absolute PMN count of at least 250 cells/mm^3 (0.25 × 10^9/L) or greater and a positive ascitic fluid bacterial culture without an obvious intra-abdominal source of infection.[44–46] Ascitic fluid diagnostic testing should be performed before treatment is initiated because even a single dose of broad-spectrum antibiotics can lead to no growth on bacterial culture in 86% of cases (**Fig. 1**).

Table 2
Indications for diagnostic paracentesis

Indicator	Examples
(1) Emergency room visit or hospital admission	—
(2) Local signs or symptoms of peritonitis	Abdominal pain or tenderness, vomiting, diarrhea, paralytic ileus
(3) Systemic signs or symptoms of infection	Fever, hypotension, leukocytosis, acidosis, hypothermia
(4) HE	—
(5) Renal failure	—
(6) Worsening of liver function	—

Data from Runyon BA, AASLD. Introduction to the revised American Association for the Study of Liver Diseases Practice Guideline management of adult patients with ascites due to cirrhosis 2012. Hepatology 2013;57:1651–3.

Distinguishing from secondary bacterial peritonitis

The fluid PMN count in secondary bacterial peritonitis is characteristically at least 250 cells/mm^3 (usually thousands) and multiple organisms, including fungi, are identified on Gram stain and culture. Laboratory diagnostic criteria for secondary bacterial peritonitis includes 2 of the following: ascitic fluid protein greater than 1 g/dL, lactate

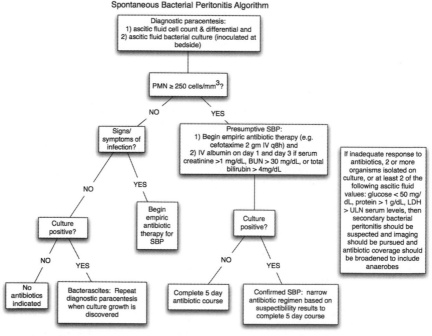

Fig. 1. Algorithm approach to SBP diagnosis and treatment. BUN, blood urea nitrogen; LDH, lactate dehydrogenase; PMN, polymorphonuclear leukocyte; SBP, spontaneous bacterial peritonitis; ULN, upper limit of normal. (*Data from* Runyon BA, AASLD. Introduction to the revised American Association for the Study of Liver Diseases Practice Guideline management of adult patients with ascites caused by/because of cirrhosis 2012. Hepatology 2013;57:1651–3.)

dehydrogenase higher than the upper limit of normal for serum, and glucose less than 50 mg/dL. In addition, ascitic fluid carcinoembryonic antigen greater than 5 ng/mL and alkaline phosphatase greater than 240 U/L have been shown to be associated with gut perforation.[10,47]

Criteria for treatment

Patients with suspected SBP and ascitic fluid PMN greater than or equal to 250 cells/mm^3 (0.25 × 10^9/L) should receive empiric antibiotic therapy.[45] An asymptomatic patient with bacterascites (normal ascitic PMN count defined as less than 250 cells/mm^3 and positive ascitic fluid culture) does not require immediate antibiotic treatment because bacterascites usually represents transient colonization. In this situation, the patient should undergo a follow-up paracentesis when the culture growth is discovered to repeat the cell count and culture results to ensure that bacterascites has not progressed to true SBP. However, any cirrhotic patient with concerning signs or symptoms that may indicate infection, such as fever (temperature greater than 37.8°C or 100°F), abdominal pain, or unexplained HE, should begin empiric antibiotic treatment of SBP, regardless of ascitic fluid PMN count (**Fig. 1**).[3,42]

Treatment regimens

Broad-spectrum antibiotic therapy is recommended for treatment of proven or suspected SBP and may be narrowed when susceptibility results become available

Table 3
SBP therapy and special considerations

Special Considerations	Antibiotic Therapy	Reasonable Alternative
Standard therapy	Cefotaxime 2 g IV q8 h × 5 d	Ceftriaxone 1 g IV q12 h or 2 g IV q24 h × 5 d
Uncomplicated SBP[a]	Ofloxacin 400 mg PO bid × 8 d is an option	Similar widely bioavailable fluoroquinolone (eg, ciprofloxacin 500 mg PO bid or levofloxacin 500 mg PO q24 h)
Nosocomial SBP	Extended spectrum antibiotics (eg, carbapenems, piperacillin/tazobactam)	Depends on local resistance patterns
Fluoroquinolone or trimethoprim/ sulfamethoxazole SBP prophylaxis	Cefotaxime 2 mg IV q8 h × 5 d	Similar third-generation cephalosporin (eg, ceftriaxone 1–2 g IV q24 h)
β-Lactam hypersensitivity	Ciprofloxacin 400 mg IV q12 h	Levofloxacin 750 mg IV q24 h
Advanced liver or renal failure: serum creatinine greater than 1 mg/dL, blood urea nitrogen greater than 30 mg/dL, or total bilirubin greater than 4 mg/dL	IV cefotaxime 2 g IV q8 h × 5 d *plus* IV albumin 1.5 g/kg given on day 1 and 1.0 g/kg given on day 3	—

Abbreviations: bid, twice a day; IV, intravenous; PO, by mouth; q, every.
   [a] Community-acquired SBP with absence of shock, ileus, gastrointestinal hemorrhage, greater than grade 2 HE, and serum creatinine greater than 3 mg/dL.
   Data from Runyon BA, AASLD. Introduction to the revised American Association for the Study of Liver Diseases Practice Guideline management of adult patients with ascites due to cirrhosis 2012. Hepatology 2013;57:1651–3.

(**Table 3**). Cefotaxime (2 g intravenously every 8 hours) or similar third-generation cephalosporin for a total course of 5 days is the treatment of choice.[48–51] Oral oflox-acin (400 mg by mouth twice a day for an average of 8 days) has been shown in one randomized controlled trial to be as effective as intravenous (IV) cefotaxime for hospi-talized patients with SBP without vomiting, shock, grade II or greater HE, or serum creatinine greater than 3 mg/dL.[52] Ciprofloxacin (400 mg IV twice a day) or levofloxa-cin (750 mg IV every 24 hours) can be used in patients who have a penicillin allergy, but should be avoided in patients who have been receiving a fluoroquinolone for SBP pro-phylaxis. Extended spectrum antibiotics, such as carbapenems, may even be consid-ered in nosocomial cases.

Adjunctive IV albumin

In a randomized controlled study involving cirrhotic patients with SBP, the use of IV albumin (1.5 g/kg given within 6 hours of enrollment and repeated as a 1.0 g/kg dose on day 3) as an adjunctive to cefotaxime was shown to decrease in-hospital mortality compared with the use of cefotaxime alone (29% vs 10%) (**Fig. 2**).[53] Use of IV albumin should be reserved for patients with a serum creatinine greater than 1 mg/dL, blood urea nitrogen greater than 30 mg/dL, or total bilirubin greater than 4 mg/dL.[54]

Secondary prophylaxis of SBP

After a primary episode of SBP, the recurrence rate at 1 year is approximately 70%, with a 1-year overall survival rate of 30% to 50% in patients who do not receive anti-biotic prophylaxis. Secondary antibiotic prophylaxis in a cirrhotic patient with a prior history of SBP reduces the risk of SBP recurrence from 68% to 20%.[55] Most experts therefore recommend daily long-term antimicrobial prophylaxis for patients with a his-tory of one or more episodes of SBP (**Table 4**).

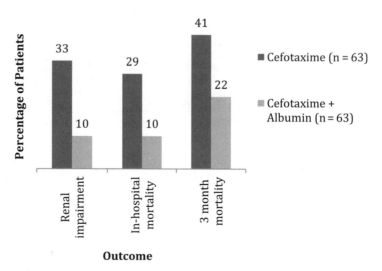

(*P* values: renal impairment *P* = .002, in-hospital mortality *P* = .01,
3 month mortality *P* = .03)

Fig. 2. Treatment with IV albumin in addition to cefotaxime prevents renal impairment and improves mortality in the setting of SBP. (*Data from* Sort P, Navasa M, Arroyo V, et al. Effect of intravenous albumin on renal impairment and mortality in patients with cirrhosis and spontaneous bacterial peritonitis. N Engl J Med 1999;341:405.)

Table 4 Indications for SBP prophylaxis	
Indicator	**Comments**
(1) Prior episode(s) of SBP	Indefinite duration unless ascites resolves
(2) Advanced liver disease without prior history of SBP	Ascitic fluid total protein less than 1.5 g/dL, and at least 2 of the following: serum creatinine ≥1.2 mg/dL, blood urea nitrogen ≥25 mg/dL, serum sodium ≤130 mEq/L or Child-Pugh ≥9 points with bilirubin ≥3 mg/dL
(3) Acute gastrointestinal bleeding	Duration limited to 7 d

Data from Runyon BA, AASLD. Introduction to the revised American Association for the Study of Liver Diseases Practice Guideline management of adult patients with ascites due to cirrhosis 2012. Hepatology 2013;57:1651–3.

Primary prophylaxis of SBP

Cirrhotic patients with low-protein ascites (less than 1.0 g/dL) and/or high serum bilirubin levels (greater than 2.5 mg/dL) are at increased risk of developing SBP.[56,57] Patients who consistently have ascitic fluid total protein less than 1.5 g/dL, and at least one of the following may be considered for long-term antibiotic prophylaxis (see **Table 4**): impaired renal function (serum creatinine greater than or equal to 1.2 mg/dL, blood urea nitrogen greater than or equal to 25 mg/dL, or serum sodium less than or equal to 130 mEq/L) or liver failure (Child-Pugh greater than or equal to 9 points, or bilirubin greater than or equal to 3 mg/dL).[3]

Primary and secondary SBP prophylaxis

Oral norfloxacin 400 mg daily has been shown to prevent spontaneous bacterial peritonitis in those with low-protein ascites and those with previous history of SBP.[55,58] Alternative regimens include oral double-strength trimethoprim-sulfamethoxazole 5 doses per week or oral ciprofloxacin 750 mg once a week,[59,60] but intermittent dosing may select for resistance.[61] Prophylaxis should be reserved for patients at high risk of developing SBP and daily dosing regimens are preferred. Reasonable alternatives include trimethoprim-sulfamethoxazole 1 double-strength tablet daily, ciprofloxacin 500 mg by mouth daily, or levofloxacin 250 mg by mouth daily, if norfloxacin is unavailable (**Table 5**).

Gastrointestinal hemorrhage

Between 25% and 65% of cirrhotic patients with gastrointestinal bleeding develop subsequent bacterial infection, including SBP.[62] Antibiotic prophylaxis in this setting has been shown to decrease the risk of bacterial infections, the risk of rebleeding, and overall mortality.[63]

Infection prophylaxis after gastrointestinal hemorrhage

Oral norfloxacin 400 mg twice daily for 7 days or IV ofloxacin 400 mg daily has been shown to prevent infection in patients with gastrointestinal hemorrhage.[64,65] In addition, ceftriaxone 1 g IV daily for 7 days has been shown to be superior to norfloxacin for the prevention of infection in a randomized trial in patients with 2 of the following: ascites, severe malnutrition, encephalopathy, or bilirubin greater than 3 mg/dL.[66] Thus, most experts prefer the use of IV ceftriaxone for infection prophylaxis after gastrointestinal hemorrhage in those patients with more advanced liver disease (see **Table 5**).

Table 5 SBP therapies			
Indication	Preferred Therapy	Alternative Agents	Duration
(1) Secondary SBP prophylaxis	Norfloxacin 400 mg PO daily	Double-strength trimethoprim/ sulfamethoxazole 1 tablet daily Ciprofloxacin 500 mg PO daily Levofloxacin 250 mg PO daily	Indefinite as long as ascites is present
(2) Primary SBP prophylaxis reserved for patients with advanced liver disease[a]	Norfloxacin 400 mg PO daily	Double-strength trimethoprim/ sulfamethoxazole 1 tablet daily Ciprofloxacin 500 mg PO daily Levofloxacin 250 mg PO daily	Indefinite as long as ascites is present
(3) Acute gastrointestinal hemorrhage	Ceftriaxone 1 g IV daily (preferred in patients with advanced liver disease[b])	May transition to oral therapy once patient is stabilized: Norfloxacin 400 mg PO bid Ciprofloxacin or 500 mg PO bid (or 400 mg IV bid)	7 d

[a] Ascitic fluid total protein less than 1.5 g/dL, and at least 2 of the following: serum creatinine greater than or equal to 1.2 mg/dL, blood urea nitrogen greater than or equal to 25 mg/dL, serum sodium less than or equal to 130 mEq/L or Child-Pugh greater than or equal to 9 points with bilirubin greater than or equal to 3 mg/dL.
[b] Ascites, severe malnutrition, encephalopathy, or bilirubin greater than 3 mg/dL.
  Data from Runyon BA, AASLD. Introduction to the revised American Association for the Study of Liver Diseases Practice Guideline management of adult patients with ascites due to cirrhosis 2012. Hepatology 2013;57:1651–3.

Dilutional Hyponatremia

Vasodilatation in cirrhosis triggers activation of the renin-angiotensin system and sympathetic nervous system, which leads to avid sodium and water retention with increased antidiuretic hormone release, resulting in dilutional hyponatremia. Up to 50% of patients with cirrhosis and ascites have a serum sodium concentration less than 135 mmol/L.[67] Hyponatremia is an independent risk factor for mortality in patients with cirrhosis and has been proposed as an addition to the MELD score for liver transplant prioritization.[29,68,69] Treatment specifically for hyponatremia is not necessary unless the serum sodium concentration decreases to less than 120 mmol/L, which occurs in only 1% of patients, or if there are neurologic symptoms attributed to hyponatremia. Relative fluid restriction (1000–1500 mL free water per day) and discontinuation of diuretics should be the first line of treatment in that setting.

Hepatorenal Syndrome

Approximately 20% of hospitalized patients with cirrhosis and ascites will develop some type of renal dysfunction. In 1 study, over the course of a mean follow-up of 41 months, 7.6% of hospitalized patients with ascites and cirrhosis developed hepatorenal syndrome (HRS).[70]

Diagnostic criteria for HRS

The diagnostic criteria for HRS are listed in **Box 4**.[71] There are 2 types of HRS.

- Type-1 HRS is characterized by rapidly progressive renal failure with a doubling in the initial serum creatinine to a level greater than 2.5 mg/dL (or 50% reduction in the initial 24-hour creatinine clearance to a level less than 20 mL/min) in less than 2 weeks. It is frequently triggered by a precipitating event, such as SBP, urinary tract infection, or intravascular volume contraction, and is associated with acute rapid deterioration of circulatory function with hypotension and activation of endogenous vasoconstrictor systems. Type 1 HRS leads to a poor prognosis, with a median survival of around 2 weeks in untreated patients.[72] Management is focused on the treatment of the precipitating event, the renal failure, and the systemic inflammatory response syndrome.[73] Diuretics should be discontinued and vasoconstrictors are used to decrease systemic vasodilatation and improve renal perfusion. The combination of terlipressin and albumin has been shown to be superior to albumin alone and placebo for the treatment of type 1 HRS and may be effective in more than 30% of cases.[74,75] Terlipressin is not available in the United States at this time, so midodrine, an alpha-agonist, is used instead (starting at a dose of 5–7.5 mg orally 3 times daily, titrated up to 15 mg 3 times daily), in combination with octreotide, starting with 100 μg subcutaneously 3 times daily, titrated up to 200 μg 3 times daily and albumin (up to 40 g daily in divided doses). The goal is to increase the mean arterial pressure by 15 mm Hg. This combination achieves a response rate of around 30%, as shown in case series.[76] In addition, TIPS can be used to improve renal function, but should be avoided in patients with advanced liver dysfunction. Liver transplantation is the definitive treatment of this condition, and some patients even require renal replacement therapy as a bridge to transplantation.
- Type 2 HRS is typically associated with refractory ascites and is characterized by a slower, progressive decline in renal function, typically with a serum creatinine that ranges from 1.5 to 2.5 mg/dL, and a median survival of 4 to 6 months. Treatment is centered on management of the refractory ascites, such as TIPS.

Box 4
Diagnostic criteria for hepatorenal syndrome

1. Cirrhosis with ascites

2. Serum creatinine greater than 1.5 mg/dL

3. No improvement in serum creatinine (decrease to or less than a level of 1.5 mg/dL) after at least 2 days with diuretic withdrawal and volume expansion with albumin (recommended dose is 1 g/kg body weight per day up to a maximum of 100 g per day)

4. Absence of shock

5. No current or recent treatment with nephrotoxic drugs

6. Absence of parenchymal kidney disease, as indicated by proteinuria greater than 500 mg per day, microhematuria (greater than 50 red blood cells per high-power field), and/or abnormal renal ultrasonography

Data from Salerno F, Gerbes A, Gines P, et al. Diagnosis, prevention and treatment of hepatorenal syndrome in cirrhosis. Gut 2007;56:1310–8.

Umbilical Hernia

Up to 20% of patients with cirrhosis and ascites can develop umbilical hernias.[77] Complications related to these hernias include omental or bowel strangulation, typically after paracentesis or shunt procedure, and hernia perforation. Patients should wear an abdominal binder to minimize strain and enlargement of the hernia and should be educated on the warning symptoms of an incarcerated hernia. In patients who are medical candidates for surgery (eg, Child-Turcotte-Pugh class A cirrhosis), the ascites needs to be controlled first with optimal medical management or TIPS, otherwise the hernia will recur in more than 70% of patients.[78,79]

Hepatic Hydrothorax

Approximately 5% to 10% of patients with cirrhosis and ascites develop hepatic hydrothorax, which is typically a right-sided pleural effusion. Thoracentesis does not require platelet or fresh frozen plasma transfusions, and there is no limit to the amount of fluid that can be removed.[80] Because of differences in hydrostatic pressure, the protein concentration is higher in pleural fluid than ascites. Spontaneous bacterial empyema can occur in the absence of SBP and can be treated with appropriate antibiotic therapy without placement of a chest tube.[81] Chest tube placement in patients with hepatic hydrothorax is associated with massive fluid losses, high morbidity (greater than 90%), and high mortality (greater than 30% in the absence of TIPS), so it should be avoided.[82,83] Treatment should start with dietary sodium restriction and diuretics. Therapeutic thoracentesis can be done for dyspnea. TIPS can be performed as treatment of refractory hepatic hydrothorax. Most patients with hepatic hydrothorax are not candidates for pleurodesis because of rapid reaccumulation of fluid.

VARICES
Pathophysiology and Portal Dynamics

In patients with cirrhosis, portal hypertension results from both an increase in resistance to portal blood flow and enhanced portal blood flow. The increased resistance in the liver results from architectural distortion caused by fibrosis and regenerative nodules combined with increased intrahepatic vasoconstriction caused by decreased endogenous nitric oxide production and endothelial dysfunction. In the presence of angiogenic factors and increased nitrous oxide production in the splanchnic vascular bed, splanchnic arteriolar vasodilatation and increased cardiac output increase portal venous blood inflow. Collaterals develop in response to the portal hypertension at sites of communication between the portal and systemic circulations. Compared with other collaterals, gastroesophageal varices are important because of their risk of rupture and bleeding.

Hepatic Venous Pressure Gradient

The hepatic venous pressure gradient (HVPG) is a measure of portal (sinusoidal) pressure and is obtained by catheterization of a hepatic vein via the jugular or femoral vein. The free hepatic vein pressure is subtracted from the wedged hepatic vein pressure to calculate HVPG, which is normally 3 to 5 mm Hg. An increased value indicates an intrahepatic cause of portal hypertension. The HVPG predicts the risk of developing varices and overall prognosis. An HVPG value of 10 mm Hg or greater indicates that the patient has developed clinically significant portal hypertension and varices may develop when the HVPG is greater than or equal to 10 to 12 mm Hg. The goal of therapy is to reduce the HVPG to less than 12 mm Hg or decrease by 20% from baseline values. Because of the invasive nature of the procedure and operator variability, its use for prognostic or therapeutic monitoring purposes is still not widespread in the United States.[84] It is used clinically to diagnose portal hypertension and identify the site of obstruction (prehepatic, intrahepatic, or posthepatic). It is also used to estimate the risk of liver failure following hepatic resection in patients with compensated chronic liver disease.

Indications and Methods for Variceal Screening

Varices are present in 30% to 40% of patients with compensated cirrhosis and in 60% of patients with decompensated cirrhosis at the time of diagnosis of cirrhosis.[85,86]

Variceal screening
On diagnosis of cirrhosis, screening esophagogastroduodenoscopy (EGD) is recommended to evaluate for the presence of gastroesophageal varices.[87] Less invasive markers for the presence of varices, such as platelet count, spleen size, and liver stiffness measurement, do not accurately predict the presence of varices. If no varices are found, an EGD should be repeated in 2 to 3 years. If esophageal varices are found, they are classified into 2 grades: small (less than or equal to 5 mm) and large (greater than 5 mm).[88,89]

Special circumstances
Individuals who are already on a nonselective β-blocker (NSBB) (eg, propranolol, nadolol) do not need to undergo screening EGD. Those patients taking a selective β-blocker (eg, metoprolol, atenolol) for other reasons should consider switching to a NSBB or carvedilol.

Preprimary and Primary Prophylaxis of Variceal Bleeding

Patients with compensated cirrhosis without gastroesophageal varices typically develop varices at a rate of 5% to 10% per year. In addition, patients with small esophageal varices progress to large varices at a rate of 8% per year.[86] It is important to decrease the risk of variceal hemorrhage, which occurs at a rate of 5% to 15% per year, with the highest rates in those with large varices, decompensated cirrhosis, or red wale markings on the varices.[90]

Absence of varices
No therapy can be recommended to prevent the development of varices. NSBBs do not prevent the development of varices in the absence of demonstrable effect on HVPG and are associated with unwanted side effects.[85] Individuals with compensated cirrhosis and absence of varices should undergo screening EGD every 2 to 3 years.

Small esophageal varices
In patients with small esophageal varices (5 mm or less) that have not bled, NSBBs may slow down variceal growth but have not been shown to confer a survival advantage.[91] Given the potential for side effects, the use of NSBBs for prophylaxis in those with small esophageal varices is reserved for those at higher risk of hemorrhage, namely those with red wale marks on varices or Child class B or C cirrhosis (**Table 6**). For patients not receiving prophylaxis with an NSBB, EGD should be repeated in 2 years, or at the time of hepatic decompensation, or annually for those with decompensated liver disease.

Large esophageal varices
In patients with large varices (greater than 5 mm) that have not bled, both NSBBs and endoscopic variceal ligation (EVL) reduce the incidence of first variceal hemorrhage. In a meta-analysis, EVL reduced risk of bleeding slightly more than NSBB use, but there

Table 6
Child-Turcotte-Pugh classification of cirrhosis

Parameter	Points Assigned		
	1	2	3
Encephalopathy	None	Grade 1 to 2	Grade 3 to 4
Ascites	Absent-Slight (detectable on imaging only)	Moderate (or diuretic responsive)	Severe (or diuretic-refractory)
Albumin (g/dL)	>3.5	2.8 to 3.5	<2.8
Bilirubin (mg/dL)[a]	1 to 2	2 to 3	>3
Prothrombin Time			
Seconds more than control	1 to 4	4 to 6	>6
INR	<1.7	1.8 to 2.3	>2.3

Class A (5–6 points), class B (7–9 points), and class C (10–15 points).
Abbreviation: INR, International Normalized Ratio.
a In cases of cholestatic liver disease, such as primary biliary cirrhosis and primary sclerosing cholangitis, the bilirubin points are sometimes considered differently: 1 point for 1 to 4 mg/dL, 2 points for 4 to 10 mg/dL, and 3 points for greater than 10 mg/dL.
Data from Child CI, Turcotte J. Surgery and portal hypertension. In: Child CI, editor. The liver and portal hypertension. Philadelphia: WB Saunders; 1964. p. 50; and Pugh RN, Murray-Lyon IM, Dawson JL, et al. Transection of the esophagus for bleeding esophageal varices. Br J Surg 1973;60:646–9.

was no difference in mortality and there was a risk of procedure-related complications with endoscopy.[92] NSBBs decrease cardiac output (β-1 effect) and induce splanchnic vasoconstriction (β-2 effect) to decrease venous portal blood inflow. In most of the published studies, investigators titrated the NSBBs to decrease the heart rate by 25% from baseline but, because the heart rate reduction does not correlate with HVPG reduction, most experts recommend increasing to the maximally tolerated dose or until the heart rate is approximately 55 beats per minute. There are promising data on carvedilol as a possible alternative agent that is well tolerated.[93] Patients receiving variceal prophylaxis need to continue the NSBB indefinitely, but they do not need follow-up EGD. For those who have a contraindication to or intolerance of NSBBs, EVL should be performed every 2 to 4 weeks until the varices are eradicated. After obliteration is achieved, patients need to continue with surveillance EGDs every 6 to 12 months indefinitely (**Table 7**).

Treatment of Acute Variceal Bleeding

Variceal bleeding accounts for 70% of all cases of upper gastrointestinal bleeding in patients with cirrhosis. Esophageal variceal bleeding spontaneously resolves in 40% to 50% of cases, but there is a 30% to 40% chance of early rebleeding in the first 6 weeks. Initial treatment of bleeding is effective in 80% to 90% of cases but mortality remains approximately 15% to 20%, with most deaths caused by liver failure, hepatorenal syndrome, and infections, and occurring predominantly in Child class C cirrhotic patients.[94,95] The management of variceal bleeding requires a multipronged approach (**Table 8**).

General management

Patients with suspected variceal hemorrhage should be admitted to the intensive care unit. Establishing intravenous access and providing volume resuscitation should be performed immediately to achieve hemodynamic stability. Blood transfusion should

Table 7
Primary prophylaxis against variceal hemorrhage

Regimen	Starting Dose/ Frequency	Goal	Monitoring
Propranolol	20 mg bid	Maximal tolerance or heart rate 55 bpm	Assess heart rate at every visit
Nadolol	20–40 mg once a day (adjust for renal insufficiency)	Maximal tolerance or heart rate 55 bpm	Assess heart rate at every visit
Carvedilol	6.25 mg once a day	Maximal tolerance or heart rate 55 bpm, up to a dose of 12.5 mg once a day	Assess heart rate at every visit
EVL	Every 2–4 wk	Variceal obliteration	Surveillance EGD 1–3 months after initial obliteration, then once every 6–12 mo

Abbreviation: bpm, beats per minute.
  Data from Garcia-Tsao G, Bosch J. Management of varices and variceal hemorrhage in cirrhosis. N Engl J Med 2010;362:823–32.

be restricted to a hemoglobin level of 7 g/dL or less, because excessive transfusion increases portal pressure, risk of rebleeding, and mortality.[96]

Pharmacologic therapy
A vasoconstrictor agent should be started at the time of admission and continued for 2 to 5 days. Terlipressin, a synthetic vasopressin analogue, has been shown to decrease mortality but is not widely available in the United States.[97] Instead, octreotide, a somatostatin analogue, is available in the United States. Its efficacy is controversial because it is associated with tachyphylaxis, but it may provide some benefit when used in combination with endoscopic therapy.[98]

Table 8
Treatment of acute variceal hemorrhage

Regimen	Options
General management	Admit to intensive care unit Resuscitation but limit transfusion to hemoglobin level of 7 g/dL Secure intravenous access Consider intubation and mechanical ventilation
Vasoconstrictor	IV octreotide (50 μg bolus followed by 50 μg/h infusion) for 2–5 d IV terlipressin (2 mg q4 h for first 48 h, followed by 1 mg q4 h) for 2–5 d
Antibiotic prophylaxis	IV ceftriaxone 1 g daily for 7 d (preferred in Child class B and C cirrhosis) Oral norfloxacin 400 mg bid for 7 d
Endoscopic therapy	EVL (preferred) Endoscopic variceal sclerotherapy
Salvage therapy	Balloon tamponade (only temporary, maximum 24 h) TIPS

Data from Garcia-Tsao G, Bosch J. Management of varices and variceal hemorrhage in cirrhosis. N Engl J Med 2010;362:823–32.

Endoscopic therapy

Endoscopic therapy, preferably EVL, should be performed within 12 hours of admission.[99] Sclerotherapy is an option when EVL is not technically feasible. Delaying endoscopic therapy for more than 15 hours increases mortality.

Infection prophylaxis

The use of prophylactic antibiotics (norfloxacin or ceftriaxone) decreases the rate of bacterial infection, risk of early rebleeding, and mortality.[42,66] Prophylaxis should be provided as noted earlier.

Rescue therapy

Rescue therapy is still warranted in 10% to 20% of cases because of failure to control bleeding or recurrent bleeding. Early placement of a TIPS within 24 to 48 hours after admission has been shown to improve survival in patients at high risk of rebleeding (HVPG greater than or equal to 20 mm Hg or Child class C cirrhosis).[100,101] Balloon tamponade can assist with temporary control of hemorrhage in patients with difficult to control bleeding awaiting more definitive therapy (eg, TIPS or endoscopic therapy).

Gastric varices

Gastric varices are present in 20% of patients with portal hypertension, but only account for 5% to 10% of all cases of upper gastrointestinal bleeding in cirrhotic patients. Endoscopic variceal obturation with tissue adhesive (eg, N-butyl-2-cyanoacrylate, isobutyl-2-cyanoacrylate, or thrombin) is preferred rather than EVL for initial management of bleeding.[102,103] This technique requires special endoscopic expertise so, if it is not available, TIPS can also be used to control the bleeding successfully as first-line therapy or in cases of recurrent bleeding.[104]

Secondary Prophylaxis of Variceal Bleeding

Untreated cirrhotic patients with a history of variceal bleeding have a 60% risk of rebleeding within 1 to 2 years, with a 20% risk of dying with each episode.[105] In the absence of TIPS placement, patients should be started on prophylactic therapy with an NSBB before discharge from the hospital.

Pharmacologic therapy

NSBBs reduce the variceal rebleeding rate to around 43%. The combination of an NSBB and isosorbide mononitrate may reduce the bleeding rate further, but this combination has greater side effects and is poorly tolerated.[94,106] Thus, most patients are treated with NSBBs alone.

Endoscopic therapy

EVL therapy is superior to sclerotherapy for secondary prophylaxis and decreases the rebleeding rate to around 32%.[107] Sessions should be repeated every 7 to 14 days until the varices are obliterated and then upper endoscopy repeated every 3 to 6 months for surveillance.

Combination therapy

The combination of pharmacologic and endoscopic therapy is superior to either modality alone in decreasing the rebleeding rate to 14% to 23%, although there is no statistical difference in mortality.[108–110]

Portosystemic shunt

Portosystemic shunt surgery is effective in preventing rebleeding but has no impact on survival and is associated with an increased risk of postprocedure HE. TIPS has similarly been shown to be superior to endoscopic therapy and pharmacologic therapy in reducing the risk of rebleeding but with no difference in mortality, an increased risk of HE, and increased costs.[111] TIPS should be reserved for Child class A and B cirrhotic patients who fail the combination of pharmacologic and endoscopic therapy.

HE
Clinical Features

HE is the result of hepatic insufficiency from acute liver failure or cirrhosis, or from portosystemic shunting, even in the absence of intrinsic liver disease. It can present with a broad range of neuropsychiatric abnormalities and varying severity. The pathogenesis of this condition is not well defined. Accumulation of ammonia from the gut and other sources because of impaired hepatic clearance or portosystemic shunting can lead to accumulation of glutamine in brain astrocytes, leading to swelling. This condition can be aggravated by hyponatremia.[112] Other mediators may also play a role.

Diagnosis and Classification

There is no consensus on the diagnostic criteria for HE. Diagnosis requires the exclusion of other causes of altered mental status (**Box 5**). Overt HE consists of neurologic and psychiatric abnormalities that can be detected by bedside clinical tests, whereas minimal HE can only be distinguished by specific psychometric tests, because these patients have normal mental and neurologic status on clinical examination. Overt HE occurs in at least 30% to 45% of patients with cirrhosis and in 10% to 50% of patients with TIPS.[113]

Clinical Presentation

The clinical diagnosis of overt HE is based on the combination of (1) impaired mental status, which is commonly graded by the West Haven Criteria (**Table 9**); and (2) impaired neuromotor function, such as hyperreflexia, hypertonicity, and asterixis.[114] Patients with HE may present with alterations in intellectual, cognitive, emotional, behavioral, psychomotor, and fine motor skills. These alterations can lead to

---

Box 5
Alternative causes of altered mental status to consider in patients with suspected HE

Hypoxia

Hypercapnia

Acidosis

Uremia

Medications or intoxication

Electrolyte disturbances

Central nervous system abnormalities (eg, seizure, stroke, intracerebral hemorrhage, meningitis)

Hypoglycemia

Delirium tremens

Wernicke-Korsakoff syndrome

Delirium

Data from Prakash R, Mullen KD. Mechanisms, diagnosis and management of hepatic encephalopathy. Nat Rev Gastroenterol Hepatol 2010;7:515–25.

Table 9
West Haven Criteria for semiquantitative grading of mental state

Grade	Criteria
1	Trivial lack of awareness Euphoria or anxiety Shortened attention span Impaired performance of addition
2	Lethargy or apathy Minimal disorientation of time or place Subtle personality changes Inappropriate behavior
3	Somnolence to semistupor but responsive to verbal stimuli Confusion Gross disorientation
4	Coma (unresponsive to verbal or noxious stimuli)

Data from Ferenci P, Lockwood A, Mullen K, et al. Hepatic encephalopathy–definition, nomenclature, diagnosis, and quantification: final report of the working party at the 11th World Congresses of Gastroenterology, Vienna, 1998. Hepatology 2002;35:716–21.

personality changes, decreased energy level, impaired sleep-wake cycle, impaired cognition, diminished consciousness, asterixis, or loss of motor control. Although patients with HE may develop focal neurologic findings, such as hemiplegia, an alternative cause for a new focal neurologic deficit (eg, intracerebral hemorrhage) should be investigated further.

Diagnostic Tests

HE is a diagnosis of exclusion of other causes of altered mental status. Precipitating factors for HE should be explored concurrently.

Laboratory testing

Although arterial and venous ammonia levels correlate with the severity of HE up to a certain point, the blood sample has be to collected without the use of a tourniquet and must be transported on ice to the laboratory to be analyzed within 20 minutes to ensure accuracy of the results.[115,116] In addition, there are many nonhepatic causes of hyperammonemia, such as gastrointestinal bleeding, renal failure, hypovolemia, extensive muscle use, urea cycle disorder, parenteral nutrition, urosepsis, and the use of certain drugs (eg, valproic acid). Although patients with HE have increased serum ammonia levels, the severity of HE does not correlate with serum ammonia levels beyond a certain point. Serial ammonia levels are not routinely used to follow patients, because the clinical presentation and clinical response to treatment are most important.

Neuropsychometric tests

In the absence of obvious physical examination findings of HE, neuropsychometric tests can be used to identify disturbances in attention, visuospatial abilities, fine motor skills, and memory.[117] These neuropsychometric tests are helping in identifying minimal HE, which may be associated with impaired driving skills. However, many of these tests require special expertise, can be time-consuming to administer, and may not be widely available for use in the United States. The most commonly performed test is the number connection tests, which can be quickly and easily administered in the office or at the bedside, although specificity is limited.

General Approach to the Management of HE

In addition to excluding other causes of altered mentation, the management of acute HE should focus on providing supportive care, identifying and treating any precipitating causes (**Box 6**, **Table 10**), reducing nitrogenous load in the gut, and assessing the need for long-term therapy and liver transplant evaluation.

Correction of precipitating factors

Among the precipitating factors for HE, common categories include (1) increased nitrogen load (eg, gastrointestinal bleed, infection, excess dietary protein), (2) decreased toxin clearance (eg, hypovolemia, renal failure, constipation, portosystemic shunt, medication noncompliance, acute-on-chronic liver failure), and (3) altered neurotransmission (eg, sedating medication, alcohol, hypoxia, hypoglycemia).[118]

Acute HE

Approximately 70% to 80% of patients with overt HE improve after correction of these precipitating factors. Patients with grade 3 or higher HE may need to be managed in an intensive care or step-down unit, with consideration of intubation for airway protection if needed.

Prevention of recurrent HE

Once patients show clinical improvement, management then transitions to the prevention of recurrent HE, including reinforcement of compliance with treatment. Therapy for HE may be discontinued if a precipitant is identified and appropriately managed in patients who do not have a prior history of overt HE.

Medical Therapy for HE

Rapid response to first-line medical therapy supports the diagnosis of HE. Most patients respond within 24 to 48 hours of initiation of treatment. Prolongation of symptoms beyond 72 hours despite attempts at treatment should prompt further

---

Box 6
Evaluation and management of altered mental status and acute overt HE in cirrhotic patients

1. Assess for non-HE causes of altered mental status, such as delirium, intoxication, alcohol withdrawal, and hypoglycemia. Consider noncontrast computed tomography scan head to assess for acute intracranial process if new focal neurologic findings are found.

2. Assess for clinical and neurologic examination findings consistent with HE: somnolence, hyperreflexia, asterixis, and posturing. Grade HE severity by West Haven Criteria or Glasgow Coma Scale.

3. Triage for patient safety: consider hospital admission for grade 2 HE and monitoring in intensive care unit or step-down unit for grade 3 or higher HE. Consider intubation if patient is unable to protect airway.

4. Assess for precipitating causes of HE and treat accordingly if found: thorough interview and physical examination, laboratory tests (eg, electrolytes, glucose, renal function, cell counts, cultures, urine drug screen, stool for *Clostridium difficile*), and imaging (eg, chest radiograph).

5. Treat HE with lactulose (per oral, nasogastric tube, or rectum) with or without rifaximin.

6. Assess need for long-term therapy for prevention of recurrent HE.

7. Assess need for liver transplant evaluation.

Data from Bajaj JS. Review article: the modern management of hepatic encephalopathy. Aliment Pharmacol Ther 2010;31:537–47.

Table 10
Precipitating causes of HE, diagnostic tests, and treatments

Precipitating Cause	Diagnostic Tests	Treatment
Increased Nitrogen Load		
Gastrointestinal hemorrhage	Stool analysis, nasogastric tube	Endoscopic or angiographic therapy, blood transfusion, antibiotic prophylaxis
Infections	Appropriate blood and fluid cultures, chest radiograph, skin examination	Antibiotic therapy
Electrolyte disturbances	Metabolic panel	Correct hyponatremia, hyperkalemia, or hypokalemia
Surgery		
Excess dietary protein	—	Avoid protein restriction, which may be harmful. Consider oral branched chain amino acids in patients with poor protein tolerance
Decreased Toxin Clearance		
Hypotension or hypovolemia	Blood pressure, serum blood urea nitrogen/creatinine, urine tests	Fluid resuscitation, albumin, discontinue diuretics, limit paracenteses, control diarrhea
Renal failure	Serum blood urea nitrogen/creatinine, urine tests	Discontinue diuretics and nephrotoxic medications
Constipation, bowel obstruction, or ileus	History, abdominal imaging	Laxative or enema for constipation
Poor compliance with medical therapy	History	Lactulose ± rifaximin
Portosystemic shunt	History, imaging	Closure of shunt or obliteration of large collaterals (reserved for severe, persistent HE)
Acute on Chronic Liver Failure		
Development of hepatocellular carcinoma	Imaging	—
Vascular occlusion or thrombosis	Imaging	—
Altered Neurotransmission		
Psychoactive medications or toxins	History, urine drug screen	Discontinue benzodiazepines, narcotics, and other sedating medications; discontinue alcohol use
Hypoglycemia	Serum glucose	Glucose
Hypoxia	Oxygen saturation, arterial blood gas	Oxygen supplementation

Data from Mullen KD. Review of the final report of the 1998 Working Party on definition, nomenclature and diagnosis of hepatic encephalopathy. Aliment Pharmacol Ther 2007;25 Suppl 1:11–6.

investigation for other causes of altered mentation. Patients should receive empiric therapy for HE while being assessed for alternative causes of altered mental status and identifying precipitating causes (**Box 7**, see **Table 10**). Treatment of acute overt HE should be followed by prevention of secondary HE.

Nonabsorbable disaccharides

Nonabsorbable disaccharides, such as lactulose, are considered the first-line treatment of HE.[119–121] Lactulose is metabolized by bacteria in the colon to acetic and lactic acid, which decrease colonic pH, decrease survival of urease-producing bacteria in the gut, and facilitates conversion of NH_3 to NH_4^+, which is less readily absorbed by the gut. The cathartic effect of these agents also increases fecal nitrogen waste. A meta-analysis showed no survival benefit of nonabsorbable disaccharides and inferiority compared with antibiotics for the management of HE, but there was significant heterogeneity across the trials, with variable end points and small sample sizes.[122] Although the effectiveness of nonabsorbable disaccharides in the management of HE remains controversial, extensive clinical experience supports use of this therapy. An open-label, randomized, controlled, single-center study showed that lactulose is more effective than placebo in the prevention of secondary overt HE.[123] For acute overt HE, the usual starting oral dose of lactulose is 10 to 30 g (15–45 mL) every 1 to 2 hours until

---

Box 7
Therapies for overt HE

Acute/episodic HE

1. Supportive care, airway protection.

2. Identification and treatment of precipitating causes.

3. Lactulose 10 to 30 g by mouth/nasogastric tube every 1 to 2 hours until bowel movement, then 10 to 30 g by mouth 2 to 4 times daily, titrated to 2 to 3 soft stools daily; or lactulose enema (300 mL in 1 L water) every 6 to 8 hours until able to oral form.

4. Rifaximin 550 mg by mouth twice daily.

5. Do not limit protein intake.

6. Consider need for long-term management of HE and liver transplant evaluation.

Recurrent or persistent HE

1. Avoidance and prevention of precipitating factors.

2. Lactulose 10 to 30 g by mouth 2 to 4 times daily, titrated to 2 to 3 soft stools daily.

3. Rifaximin 550 mg by mouth twice daily.

4. Maintain protein intake of 1.0 to 1.5 g/kg daily, over 4 to 6 meals daily with nighttime snack. Vegetable-based protein is preferred for patients with severe persistent HE. Oral branched-chain amino acid supplementation may be considered in those who are intolerant of protein.

5. For severe persistent HE, some patients may be considered for closure or reduction of TIPS diameter or occlusion/embolization of larger portosystemic collaterals (not commonly done in the United States).

6. Liver transplant referral for appropriate candidates.

Data from Garcia-Tsao G, Lim JK; Members of Veterans Affairs Hepatitis CRCP. Management and treatment of patients with cirrhosis and portal hypertension: recommendations from the Department of Veterans Affairs Hepatitis C Resource Center Program and the National Hepatitis C Program. Am J Gastroenterol 2009;104:1802–29.

a bowel movement occurs, then adjust to 10 to 30 g (15–45 mL) 2 to 4 times daily, titrated to induce 2 to 3 soft bowel movements daily. This dose may be continued indefinitely for those with recurrent or persistent HE. For comatose patients, the medication can be administered through a nasogastric tube or rectally as an enema (300 mL in 1 L of water ever 6–8 hours) until the patient is awake enough to start oral therapy.

Antibiotics

Rifaximin is a minimally absorbed (less than 0.4%) antibiotic with broad-spectrum in vitro activity against gram-positive and gram-negative aerobic and anaerobic bacteria. In a large multicenter trial, rifaximin (550 mg twice daily) with lactulose maintained remission from HE better than lactulose alone and also reduced the number of hospitalizations involving HE.[124] Neomycin (1–4 g daily in divided doses) and metronidazole (starting dose 250 mg twice daily) have been used to treat HE in the past, but, because of concerns of toxicity and side effects, rifaximin is now the preferred antibiotic.[114]

Nutrition

Dietary protein restriction is not advised for the management of HE because loss of skeletal muscle, which metabolizes ammonia, can lead to worsening HE.[125] Thus, patients with cirrhosis are recommended to consume a high-protein diet of at least 1.0 g/kg to 1.5 g/kg daily.[126] Eating 4 to 6 small meals daily with a nighttime snack may help avoid protein loading.

HEPATOCELLULAR CARCINOMA

Patients with cirrhosis are at risk for developing hepatocellular carcinoma (HCC). The highest risk of HCC is in those with hereditary hemochromatosis, chronic hepatitis B, and chronic hepatitis C, with incidence rates estimated at around 2% to 8% per year.[127–129] In the United States, hepatitis C with cirrhosis is the most common cause of HCC. The prognosis for patients diagnosed with HCC is typically poor, with an estimated median survival of 4.3 to 20 months and a 5-year survival of 10% to 15%, which decreases further to 0% to 10% when HCC is detected after onset of symptoms.

HCC Surveillance

In patients with cirrhosis, the American Association for the Study of Liver Disease (AASLD) recommends ultrasound examination every 6 months for HCC surveillance.[128] Ultrasound imaging has a sensitivity of 65% to 80% and a specificity of 87% to 94% for detecting HCC, but the technique is operator dependent. Dynamic contrast-enhanced computed tomography (CT) scan and magnetic resonance imaging (MRI) are not used for routine surveillance but can be performed as secondary tests for nodules detected on ultrasound. There is controversy regarding the use of serum alphafetoprotein monitoring because of its low sensitivity and specificity; it should not be used alone for HCC surveillance.

HCC Diagnosis

The diagnosis of HCC for lesions greater than 1 cm can be made without need for a liver biopsy if typical imaging features on dynamic contrast-enhanced CT scan or MRI are present. These features include early arterial enhancement and delayed washout in the venous or delayed phase. Lesions less than 1 cm should be followed with imaging at 3-month intervals. Image-guided biopsy or close monitoring should be considered for atypical lesions.

HCC Treatment

Hepatic resection is considered a treatment option for patients with HCC and compensated cirrhosis without significant portal hypertension, but more than 50% develop recurrence of HCC within 5 years.[128,130] The same risk of recurrent HCC results from locoregional therapy, such as radiofrequency ablation, percutaneous ethanol injection, and chemoembolization. Patients with HCC who meet Milan criteria (solitary HCC lesion less than 5 cm or up to 3 nodules smaller than 3 cm) and have no radiographic evidence of extrahepatic disease, but who are not candidates for surgical resection, are considered liver transplantation candidates and granted priority for liver transplantation. The 1-year and 5-year posttransplant survival rates for patients with tumors meeting Milan criteria are 89% and 61%, respectively, which are considered acceptable rates.[131] Certain transplant centers in the United States have expanded transplant criteria (HCC that exceeds Milan criteria or downstaging of HCC through neoadjuvant locoregional therapy to within the Milan criteria) that may provide a patient consideration for transplantation under investigational or specialized protocols.

LIVER TRANSPLANTATION
Indications for Liver Transplantation

Liver transplantation is a lifesaving surgery for patients with acute and chronic liver diseases. The major disorders that may result in consideration for liver transplantation include acute liver failure, chronic liver disease with advanced cirrhosis, HCC, and liver-based metabolic defects. In 2012, more than 6000 liver transplants were performed in the United States, and chronic hepatitis C virus infection was the most common indication for the transplantation. Advances in transplantation have improved posttransplant survival rates in the United States to 87.7% at 1 year after liver transplantation, 79.9% at 3 years, and 74.3% at 5 years.[132]

Timing for Liver Transplantation

When considering referral for liver transplantation, the natural history of the disease should be compared against the expected survival after transplantation. Because the transplant evaluation may take weeks to months to complete, for patients who have an indication for liver transplantation, it is ideal to refer them early in the clinical course rather than late. In addition, patients diagnosed with hepatopulmonary syndrome or portopulmonary hypertension, attributed to cirrhosis, or a new diagnosis of HCC should be referred for consideration of transplantation.

Use of prognostic scoring systems

Scoring systems initially designed to predict outcome following portocaval shunt surgery and TIPS have been used to predict overall survival in patients with cirrhosis.[133–135] The Child-Turcotte-Pugh (CTP) classification (see **Table 6**) can be used to predict short-term prognosis (**Table 11**) in patients awaiting transplantation.[136–138] Patients with CTP score 7 to 9 (class B) have an estimated 1-year survival of 80%. In the past, a CTP score of 7 or greater was considered a minimal listing criterion for liver transplantation.[139] The MELD score has been shown to be a useful tool in predicting short-term survival in patients with chronic liver disease.[140] The modified version uses a continuous scale from 6 to 40, based on serum bilirubin, international normalized ratio of prothrombin time (INR), and serum creatinine. It has been shown to predict mortality for patients on the liver transplant waiting list and was implemented in February 2002, replacing CTP score, to prioritize patients for donor allocation in the United States.[141,142] Based on current

Table 11
Modified CTP classification of severity of cirrhosis and corresponding estimated short-term survival

CTP Class	CTP Score	1-y % Survival	2-y % Survival
A	5 to 6	95	90
B	7 to 9	80	70
C	10 to 15	45	38

Data from D'Amico G, Garcia-Tsao G, Pagliaro L. Natural history and prognostic indicators of survival in cirrhosis: a systematic review of 118 studies. J Hepatol 2006;44:217–31.

guidelines, a patient with a MELD score of 10 or greater or a CTP score of 7 or greater should be referred to a liver transplant center for evaluation.[143]

Decompensated cirrhosis

The development of decompensated cirrhosis, defined by the occurrence of a complication, such as ascites, variceal bleeding, HE, SBP, or hepatorenal syndrome, also negatively influences prognosis. In a natural history study in patients with cirrhosis, more than 90% of the patients who remained compensated were still alive at 5 years, compared with only 50% survival at 5 years among those who experienced a decompensating event.[1] Moreover, once decompensation occurred, 20% died within 1 year. Similar findings have been repeated in other studies.[144–146] Patients therefore should be referred for transplant evaluation when they experience their first major cirrhosis-related complication, such as ascites, variceal bleeding, or HE.

SUMMARY

Patients with cirrhosis who experience hepatic decompensation, such as the development of ascites, SBP, variceal hemorrhage, or hepatic encephalopathy, or who develop HCC, are at a higher risk of mortality. Management should be focused on the prevention of recurrence of complications, and these patients should be referred for consideration of liver transplantation.

REFERENCES

1. Gines P, Quintero E, Arroyo V, et al. Compensated cirrhosis: natural history and prognostic factors. Hepatology 1987;7:122–8.
2. Asrani SK, Larson JJ, Yawn B, et al. Underestimation of liver-related mortality in the United States. Gastroenterology 2013;145:375–82.e2.
3. Runyon BA, AASLD. Introduction to the revised American Association for the Study of Liver Diseases Practice Guideline management of adult patients with ascites due to cirrhosis 2012. Hepatology 2013;57:1651–3.
4. Planas R, Montoliu S, Balleste B, et al. Natural history of patients hospitalized for management of cirrhotic ascites. Clin Gastroenterol Hepatol 2006;4:1385–94.
5. Runyon BA, Montano AA, Akriviadis EA, et al. The serum-ascites albumin gradient is superior to the exudate-transudate concept in the differential diagnosis of ascites. Ann Intern Med 1992;117:215–20.
6. Runyon BA. Paracentesis of ascitic fluid. A safe procedure. Arch Intern Med 1986;146:2259–61.
7. Grabau CM, Crago SF, Hoff LK, et al. Performance standards for therapeutic abdominal paracentesis. Hepatology 2004;40:484–8.

8. Runyon BA, Canawati HN, Akriviadis EA. Optimization of ascitic fluid culture technique. Gastroenterology 1988;95:1351–5.
9. Runyon BA, Antillon MR, Akriviadis EA, et al. Bedside inoculation of blood culture bottles with ascitic fluid is superior to delayed inoculation in the detection of spontaneous bacterial peritonitis. J Clin Microbiol 1990;28:2811–2.
10. Akriviadis EA, Runyon BA. Utility of an algorithm in differentiating spontaneous from secondary bacterial peritonitis. Gastroenterology 1990;98:127–33.
11. Runyon BA. Malignancy-related ascites and ascitic fluid "humoral tests of malignancy". J Clin Gastroenterol 1994;18:94–8.
12. Jeffries MA, Stern MA, Gunaratnam NT, et al. Unsuspected infection is infrequent in asymptomatic outpatients with refractory ascites undergoing therapeutic paracentesis. Am J Gastroenterol 1999;94:2972–6.
13. Veldt BJ, Laine F, Guillygomarc'h A, et al. Indication of liver transplantation in severe alcoholic liver cirrhosis: quantitative evaluation and optimal timing. J Hepatol 2002;36:93–8.
14. Eisenmenger WJ, Ahrens EH, Blondheim SH, et al. The effect of rigid sodium restriction in patients with cirrhosis of the liver and ascites. J Lab Clin Med 1949; 34:1029–38.
15. Perez-Ayuso RM, Arroyo V, Planas R, et al. Randomized comparative study of efficacy of furosemide versus spironolactone in nonazotemic cirrhosis with ascites. Relationship between the diuretic response and the activity of the renin-aldosterone system. Gastroenterology 1983;84:961–8.
16. Santos J, Planas R, Pardo A, et al. Spironolactone alone or in combination with furosemide in the treatment of moderate ascites in nonazotemic cirrhosis. A randomized comparative study of efficacy and safety. J Hepatol 2003;39:187–92.
17. Angeli P, Fasolato S, Mazza E, et al. Combined versus sequential diuretic treatment of ascites in non-azotaemic patients with cirrhosis: results of an open randomised clinical trial. Gut 2010;59:98–104.
18. Angeli P, Dalla Pria M, De Bei E, et al. Randomized clinical study of the efficacy of amiloride and potassium canrenoate in nonazotemic cirrhotic patients with ascites. Hepatology 1994;19:72–9.
19. Pockros PJ, Reynolds TB. Rapid diuresis in patients with ascites from chronic liver disease: the importance of peripheral edema. Gastroenterology 1986;90: 1827 33.
20. Wong F, Watson H, Gerbes A, et al. Satavaptan for the management of ascites in cirrhosis: efficacy and safety across the spectrum of ascites severity. Gut 2012; 61:108–16.
21. Serste T, Melot C, Francoz C, et al. Deleterious effects of beta-blockers on survival in patients with cirrhosis and refractory ascites. Hepatology 2010;52:1017–22.
22. Serste T, Francoz C, Durand F, et al. Beta-blockers cause paracentesis-induced circulatory dysfunction in patients with cirrhosis and refractory ascites: a crossover study. J Hepatol 2011;55:794–9.
23. Gines P, Arroyo V, Quintero E, et al. Comparison of paracentesis and diuretics in the treatment of cirrhotics with tense ascites. Results of a randomized study. Gastroenterology 1987;93:234–41.
24. Peltekian KM, Wong F, Liu PP, et al. Cardiovascular, renal, and neurohumoral responses to single large-volume paracentesis in patients with cirrhosis and diuretic-resistant ascites. Am J Gastroenterol 1997;92:394–9.
25. Tito L, Gines P, Arroyo V, et al. Total paracentesis associated with intravenous albumin management of patients with cirrhosis and ascites. Gastroenterology 1990;98:146–51.

26. Stanley MM, Ochi S, Lee KK, et al. Peritoneovenous shunting as compared with medical treatment in patients with alcoholic cirrhosis and massive ascites. Veterans Administration Cooperative Study on Treatment of Alcoholic Cirrhosis with Ascites. N Engl J Med 1989;321:1632–8.

27. Guardiola J, Xiol X, Escriba JM, et al. Prognosis assessment of cirrhotic patients with refractory ascites treated with a peritoneovenous shunt. Am J Gastroenterol 1995;90:2097–102.

28. Gines P, Arroyo V, Vargas V, et al. Paracentesis with intravenous infusion of albumin as compared with peritoneovenous shunting in cirrhosis with refractory ascites. N Engl J Med 1991;325:829–35.

29. Heuman DM, Abou-Assi SG, Habib A, et al. Persistent ascites and low serum sodium identify patients with cirrhosis and low MELD scores who are at high risk for early death. Hepatology 2004;40:802–10.

30. Baltz JG, Argo CK, Al-Osaimi AM, et al. Mortality after percutaneous endoscopic gastrostomy in patients with cirrhosis: a case series. Gastrointest Endosc 2010;72:1072–5.

31. Bernardi M, Caraceni P, Navickis RJ, et al. Albumin infusion in patients undergoing large-volume paracentesis: a meta-analysis of randomized trials. Hepatology 2012;55:1172–81.

32. Salerno F, Camma C, Enea M, et al. Transjugular intrahepatic portosystemic shunt for refractory ascites: a meta-analysis of individual patient data. Gastroenterology 2007;133:825–34.

33. Rossle M, Ochs A, Gulberg V, et al. A comparison of paracentesis and transjugular intrahepatic portosystemic shunting in patients with ascites. N Engl J Med 2000;342:1701–7.

34. Gines P, Uriz J, Calahorra B, et al. Transjugular intrahepatic portosystemic shunting versus paracentesis plus albumin for refractory ascites in cirrhosis. Gastroenterology 2002;123:1839–47.

35. Sanyal AJ, Genning C, Reddy KR, et al. The North American study for the treatment of refractory ascites. Gastroenterology 2003;124:634–41.

36. Salerno F, Merli M, Riggio O, et al. Randomized controlled study of TIPS versus paracentesis plus albumin in cirrhosis with severe ascites. Hepatology 2004;40:629–35.

37. Boyer TD, Haskal ZJ, American Association for the Study of Liver D. The role of transjugular intrahepatic portosystemic shunt (TIPS) in the management of portal hypertension: update 2009. Hepatology 2010;51:306.

38. Somberg KA, Lake JR, Tomlanovich SJ, et al. Transjugular intrahepatic portosystemic shunts for refractory ascites: assessment of clinical and hormonal response and renal function. Hepatology 1995;21:709–16.

39. Garcia-Tsao G. Spontaneous bacterial peritonitis: a historical perspective. J Hepatol 2004;41:522–7.

40. Evans LT, Kim WR, Poterucha JJ, et al. Spontaneous bacterial peritonitis in asymptomatic outpatients with cirrhotic ascites. Hepatology 2003;37:897–901.

41. Wong F, Bernardi M, Balk R, et al. Sepsis in cirrhosis: report on the 7th meeting of the International Ascites Club. Gut 2005;54:718–25.

42. Rimola A, Garcia-Tsao G, Navasa M, et al. Diagnosis, treatment and prophylaxis of spontaneous bacterial peritonitis: a consensus document. International Ascites Club. J Hepatol 2000;32:142–53.

43. Borzio M, Salerno F, Piantoni L, et al. Bacterial infection in patients with advanced cirrhosis: a multicentre prospective study. Dig Liver Dis 2001;33:41–8.

44. Hoefs JC, Canawati HN, Sapico FL, et al. Spontaneous bacterial peritonitis. Hepatology 1982;2:399–407.
45. Runyon BA, Hoefs JC. Culture-negative neutrocytic ascites: a variant of spontaneous bacterial peritonitis. Hepatology 1984;4:1209–11.
46. Runyon BA, Antillon MR. Ascitic fluid pH and lactate: insensitive and nonspecific tests in detecting ascitic fluid infection. Hepatology 1991;13:929–35.
47. Wu SS, Lin OS, Chen YY, et al. Ascitic fluid carcinoembryonic antigen and alkaline phosphatase levels for the differentiation of primary from secondary bacterial peritonitis with intestinal perforation. J Hepatol 2001;34:215–21.
48. Runyon BA, Akriviadis EA, Sattler FR, et al. Ascitic fluid and serum cefotaxime and desacetyl cefotaxime levels in patients treated for bacterial peritonitis. Dig Dis Sci 1991;36:1782–6.
49. Runyon BA, McHutchison JG, Antillon MR, et al. Short-course versus long-course antibiotic treatment of spontaneous bacterial peritonitis. A randomized controlled study of 100 patients. Gastroenterology 1991;100:1737–42.
50. Rimola A, Salmeron JM, Clemente G, et al. Two different dosages of cefotaxime in the treatment of spontaneous bacterial peritonitis in cirrhosis: results of a prospective, randomized, multicenter study. Hepatology 1995;21:674–9.
51. Ricart E, Soriano G, Novella MT, et al. Amoxicillin-clavulanic acid versus cefotaxime in the therapy of bacterial infections in cirrhotic patients. J Hepatol 2000;32:596–602.
52. Navasa M, Follo A, Llovet JM, et al. Randomized, comparative study of oral ofloxacin versus intravenous cefotaxime in spontaneous bacterial peritonitis. Gastroenterology 1996;111:1011–7.
53. Sort P, Navasa M, Arroyo V, et al. Effect of intravenous albumin on renal impairment and mortality in patients with cirrhosis and spontaneous bacterial peritonitis. N Engl J Med 1999;341:403–9.
54. Sigal SH, Stanca CM, Fernandez J, et al. Restricted use of albumin for spontaneous bacterial peritonitis. Gut 2007;56:597–9.
55. Gines P, Rimola A, Planas R, et al. Norfloxacin prevents spontaneous bacterial peritonitis recurrence in cirrhosis: results of a double-blind, placebo-controlled trial. Hepatology 1990;12:716–24.
56. Runyon BA. Low-protein-concentration ascitic fluid is predisposed to spontaneous bacterial peritonitis. Gastroenterology 1986;91:1343–6.
57. Garcia-Tsao G. Current management of the complications of cirrhosis and portal hypertension: variceal hemorrhage, ascites, and spontaneous bacterial peritonitis. Gastroenterology 2001;120:726–48.
58. Soriano G, Guarner C, Teixido M, et al. Selective intestinal decontamination prevents spontaneous bacterial peritonitis. Gastroenterology 1991;100:477–81.
59. Singh N, Gayowski T, Yu VL, et al. Trimethoprim-sulfamethoxazole for the prevention of spontaneous bacterial peritonitis in cirrhosis: a randomized trial. Ann Intern Med 1995;122:595–8.
60. Rolachon A, Cordier L, Bacq Y, et al. Ciprofloxacin and long-term prevention of spontaneous bacterial peritonitis: results of a prospective controlled trial. Hepatology 1995;22:1171–4.
61. Terg R, Llano K, Cobas SM, et al. Effects of oral ciprofloxacin on aerobic gram-negative fecal flora in patients with cirrhosis: results of short- and long-term administration, with daily and weekly dosages. J Hepatol 1998;29:437–42.
62. Deschenes M, Villeneuve JP. Risk factors for the development of bacterial infections in hospitalized patients with cirrhosis. Am J Gastroenterol 1999;94:2193–7.

63. Bernard B, Grange JD, Khac EN, et al. Antibiotic prophylaxis for the prevention of bacterial infections in cirrhotic patients with gastrointestinal bleeding: a meta-analysis. Hepatology 1999;29:1655–61.

64. Soriano G, Guarner C, Tomas A, et al. Norfloxacin prevents bacterial infection in cirrhotics with gastrointestinal hemorrhage. Gastroenterology 1992;103: 1267–72.

65. Blaise M, Pateron D, Trinchet JC, et al. Systemic antibiotic therapy prevents bacterial infection in cirrhotic patients with gastrointestinal hemorrhage. Hepatology 1994;20:34–8.

66. Fernandez J, Ruiz del Arbol L, Gomez C, et al. Norfloxacin vs ceftriaxone in the prophylaxis of infections in patients with advanced cirrhosis and hemorrhage. Gastroenterology 2006;131:1049–56 [quiz: 285].

67. Angeli P, Wong F, Watson H, et al. Hyponatremia in cirrhosis: results of a patient population survey. Hepatology 2006;44:1535–42.

68. Biggins SW, Rodriguez HJ, Bacchetti P, et al. Serum sodium predicts mortality in patients listed for liver transplantation. Hepatology 2005;41:32–9.

69. Ruf AE, Kremers WK, Chavez LL, et al. Addition of serum sodium into the MELD score predicts waiting list mortality better than MELD alone. Liver Transpl 2005; 11:336–43.

70. Montoliu S, Balleste B, Planas R, et al. Incidence and prognosis of different types of functional renal failure in cirrhotic patients with ascites. Clin Gastroenterol Hepatol 2010;8:616–22 [quiz: e80].

71. Salerno F, Gerbes A, Gines P, et al. Diagnosis, prevention and treatment of hepatorenal syndrome in cirrhosis. Gut 2007;56:1310–8.

72. Gines P, Guevara M, Arroyo V, et al. Hepatorenal syndrome. Lancet 2003;362: 1819–27.

73. Wong F. Recent advances in our understanding of hepatorenal syndrome. Nat Rev Gastroenterol Hepatol 2012;9:382–91.

74. Sanyal AJ, Boyer T, Garcia-Tsao G, et al. A randomized, prospective, double-blind, placebo-controlled trial of terlipressin for type 1 hepatorenal syndrome. Gastroenterology 2008;134:1360–8.

75. Martin-Llahi M, Pepin MN, Guevara M, et al. Terlipressin and albumin vs albumin in patients with cirrhosis and hepatorenal syndrome: a randomized study. Gastroenterology 2008;134:1352–9.

76. Esrailian E, Pantangco ER, Kyulo NL, et al. Octreotide/midodrine therapy significantly improves renal function and 30-day survival in patients with type 1 hepatorenal syndrome. Dig Dis Sci 2007;52:742–8.

77. Belghiti J, Durand F. Abdominal wall hernias in the setting of cirrhosis. Semin Liver Dis 1997;17:219–26.

78. Runyon BA, Juler GL. Natural history of repaired umbilical hernias in patients with and without ascites. Am J Gastroenterol 1985;80:38–9.

79. Triantos CK, Kehagias I, Nikolopoulou V, et al. Surgical repair of umbilical hernias in cirrhosis with ascites. Am J Med Sci 2011;341:222–6.

80. Xiol X, Castellote J, Cortes-Beut R, et al. Usefulness and complications of thoracentesis in cirrhotic patients. Am J Med 2001;111:67–9.

81. Xiol X, Castellvi JM, Guardiola J, et al. Spontaneous bacterial empyema in cirrhotic patients: a prospective study. Hepatology 1996;23:719–23.

82. Runyon BA, Greenblatt M, Ming RH. Hepatic hydrothorax is a relative contraindication to chest tube insertion. Am J Gastroenterol 1986;81:566–7.

83. Orman ES, Lok AS. Outcomes of patients with chest tube insertion for hepatic hydrothorax. Hepatol Int 2009;3:582–6.

84. Groszmann RJ, Wongcharatrawee S. The hepatic venous pressure gradient: anything worth doing should be done right. Hepatology 2004;39:280–2.
85. Groszmann RJ, Garcia-Tsao G, Bosch J, et al. Beta-blockers to prevent gastro-esophageal varices in patients with cirrhosis. N Engl J Med 2005;353:2254–61.
86. Merli M, Nicolini G, Angeloni S, et al. Incidence and natural history of small esophageal varices in cirrhotic patients. J Hepatol 2003;38:266–72.
87. Garcia-Tsao G, Sanyal AJ, Grace ND, et al, Practice Guidelines Committee of the American Association for the Study of Liver Disease, Practice Parameters Committee of the American College of Gastroenterology. Prevention and management of gastroesophageal varices and variceal hemorrhage in cirrhosis. Hepatology 2007;46:922–38.
88. de Franchis R, Pascal JP, Ancona E, et al. Definitions, methodology and therapeutic strategies in portal hypertension. A Consensus Development Workshop, Baveno, Lake Maggiore, Italy, April 5 and 6, 1990. J Hepatol 1992;15:256–61.
89. de Franchis R. Updating consensus in portal hypertension: report of the Baveno III Consensus Workshop on definitions, methodology and therapeutic strategies in portal hypertension. J Hepatol 2000;33:846–52.
90. North Italian Endoscopic Club for the S, Treatment of Esophageal V. Prediction of the first variceal hemorrhage in patients with cirrhosis of the liver and esophageal varices. A prospective multicenter study. N Engl J Med 1988;319:983–9.
91. Merkel C, Marin R, Angeli P, et al. A placebo-controlled clinical trial of nadolol in the prophylaxis of growth of small esophageal varices in cirrhosis. Gastroenterology 2004;127:476–84.
92. Gluud LL, Krag A. Banding ligation versus beta-blockers for primary prevention in oesophageal varices in adults. Cochrane Database Syst Rev 2012;(8):CD004544.
93. Tripathi D, Ferguson JW, Kochar N, et al. Randomized controlled trial of carvedilol versus variceal band ligation for the prevention of the first variceal bleed. Hepatology 2009;50:825–33.
94. D'Amico G, Pagliaro L, Bosch J. Pharmacological treatment of portal hypertension: an evidence-based approach. Semin Liver Dis 1999;19:475–505.
95. D'Amico G, De Franchis R, Cooperative Study G. Upper digestive bleeding in cirrhosis. Post-therapeutic outcome and prognostic indicators. Hepatology 2003;38:599–612.
96. Villanueva C, Colomo A, Bosch A, et al. Transfusion strategies for acute upper gastrointestinal bleeding. N Engl J Med 2013;368:11–21.
97. Ioannou G, Doust J, Rockey DC. Terlipressin for acute esophageal variceal hemorrhage. Cochrane Database Syst Rev 2003;(1):CD002147.
98. Banares R, Albillos A, Rincon D, et al. Endoscopic treatment versus endoscopic plus pharmacologic treatment for acute variceal bleeding: a meta-analysis. Hepatology 2002;35:609–15.
99. de Franchis R, Baveno VF. Revising consensus in portal hypertension: report of the Baveno V consensus workshop on methodology of diagnosis and therapy in portal hypertension. J Hepatol 2010;53:762–8.
100. Monescillo A, Martinez-Lagares F, Ruiz-del-Arbol L, et al. Influence of portal hypertension and its early decompression by TIPS placement on the outcome of variceal bleeding. Hepatology 2004;40:793–801.
101. Garcia-Pagan JC, Caca K, Bureau C, et al. Early use of TIPS in patients with cirrhosis and variceal bleeding. N Engl J Med 2010;362:2370–9.
102. Lo GH, Lai KH, Cheng JS, et al. A prospective, randomized trial of butyl cyanoacrylate injection versus band ligation in the management of bleeding gastric varices. Hepatology 2001;33:1060–4.

103. Tan PC, Hou MC, Lin HC, et al. A randomized trial of endoscopic treatment of acute gastric variceal hemorrhage: N-butyl-2-cyanoacrylate injection versus band ligation. Hepatology 2006;43:690–7.
104. Chau TN, Patch D, Chan YW, et al. "Salvage" transjugular intrahepatic portosystemic shunts: gastric fundal compared with esophageal variceal bleeding. Gastroenterology 1998;114:981–7.
105. Bosch J, Garcia-Pagan JC. Prevention of variceal rebleeding. Lancet 2003;361: 952–4.
106. Gournay J, Masliah C, Martin T, et al. Isosorbide mononitrate and propranolol compared with propranolol alone for the prevention of variceal rebleeding. Hepatology 2000;31:1239–45.
107. Laine L, Cook D. Endoscopic ligation compared with sclerotherapy for treatment of esophageal variceal bleeding. A meta-analysis. Ann Intern Med 1995;123: 280–7.
108. Lo GH, Lai KH, Cheng JS, et al. Endoscopic variceal ligation plus nadolol and sucralfate compared with ligation alone for the prevention of variceal rebleeding: a prospective, randomized trial. Hepatology 2000;32:461–5.
109. de la Pena J, Brullet E, Sanchez-Hernandez E, et al. Variceal ligation plus nadolol compared with ligation for prophylaxis of variceal rebleeding: a multicenter trial. Hepatology 2005;41:572–8.
110. Gonzalez R, Zamora J, Gomez-Camarero J, et al. Meta-analysis: combination endoscopic and drug therapy to prevent variceal rebleeding in cirrhosis. Ann Intern Med 2008;149:109–22.
111. Escorsell A, Banares R, Garcia-Pagan JC, et al. TIPS versus drug therapy in preventing variceal rebleeding in advanced cirrhosis: a randomized controlled trial. Hepatology 2002;35:385–92.
112. Prakash R, Mullen KD. Mechanisms, diagnosis and management of hepatic encephalopathy. Nat Rev Gastroenterol Hepatol 2010;7:515–25.
113. Poordad FF. Review article: the burden of hepatic encephalopathy. Aliment Pharmacol Ther 2007;25(Suppl 1):3–9.
114. Conn HO, Leevy CM, Vlahcevic ZR, et al. Comparison of lactulose and neomycin in the treatment of chronic portal-systemic encephalopathy. A double blind controlled trial. Gastroenterology 1977;72:573–83.
115. Ong JP, Aggarwal A, Krieger D, et al. Correlation between ammonia levels and the severity of hepatic encephalopathy. Am J Med 2003;114:188–93.
116. Kramer L, Tribl B, Gendo A, et al. Partial pressure of ammonia versus ammonia in hepatic encephalopathy. Hepatology 2000;31:30–4.
117. Weissenborn K, Ennen JC, Schomerus H, et al. Neuropsychological characterization of hepatic encephalopathy. J Hepatol 2001;34:768–73.
118. Blei AT, Cordoba J, Practice Parameters Committee of the American College of Gastroenterology. Hepatic encephalopathy. Am J Gastroenterol 2001;96: 1968–76.
119. Morgan MY, Hawley KE, Stambuk D. Lactitol versus lactulose in the treatment of chronic hepatic encephalopathy. A double-blind, randomised, cross-over study. J Hepatol 1987;4:236–44.
120. Morgan MY, Hawley KE. Lactitol vs. lactulose in the treatment of acute hepatic encephalopathy in cirrhotic patients: a double-blind, randomized trial. Hepatology 1987;7:1278–84.
121. Morgan MY, Alonso M, Stanger LC. Lactitol and lactulose for the treatment of subclinical hepatic encephalopathy in cirrhotic patients. A randomised, cross-over study. J Hepatol 1989;8:208–17.

122. Als-Nielsen B, Gluud LL, Gluud C. Non-absorbable disaccharides for hepatic encephalopathy: systematic review of randomised trials. BMJ 2004;328: 1046.
123. Agrawal A, Sharma BC, Sharma P, et al. Secondary prophylaxis of hepatic encephalopathy in cirrhosis: an open-label, randomized controlled trial of lactulose, probiotics, and no therapy. Am J Gastroenterol 2012;107:1043–50.
124. Bass NM, Mullen KD, Sanyal A, et al. Rifaximin treatment in hepatic encephalopathy. N Engl J Med 2010;362:1071–81.
125. Cordoba J, Lopez-Hellin J, Planas M, et al. Normal protein diet for episodic hepatic encephalopathy: results of a randomized study. J Hepatol 2004;41: 38–43.
126. Plauth M, Cabre E, Riggio O, et al. ESPEN guidelines on enteral nutrition: liver disease. Clin Nutr 2006;25:285–94.
127. Altekruse SF, McGlynn KA, Reichman ME. Hepatocellular carcinoma incidence, mortality, and survival trends in the United States from 1975 to 2005. J Clin Oncol 2009;27:1485–91.
128. Bruix J, Sherman M, American Association for the Study of Liver Disease. Management of hepatocellular carcinoma: an update. Hepatology 2011;53:1020–2.
129. El-Serag HB. Hepatocellular carcinoma. N Engl J Med 2011;365:1118–27.
130. Cha CH, Ruo L, Fong Y, et al. Resection of hepatocellular carcinoma in patients otherwise eligible for transplantation. Ann Surg 2003;238:315–21 [discussion: 21–3].
131. Pelletier SJ, Fu S, Thyagarajan V, et al. An intention-to-treat analysis of liver transplantation for hepatocellular carcinoma using organ procurement transplant network data. Liver Transpl 2009;15:859–68.
132. Annual Report of the U.S. Organ Procurement and Transplantation Network and the Scientific Registry of Transplant Recipients: transplant data 1994-2003. Rockville (MD), Richmond (VA), Ann Arbor (MI): Department of Health and Human Services, Health Resources and Service Administration, Healthcare Systems Bureau, Division of Transplantation; United Network for Organ Sharing; University Renal Research and Education Association; 2004.
133. Child CI, Turcotte J. Surgery and portal hypertension. In: Child CI, editor. The liver and portal hypertension. Philadelphia: WB Saunders; 1964. p. 50.
134. Pugh RN, Murray-Lyon IM, Dawson JL, et al. Transection of the oesophagus for bleeding oesophageal varices. Br J Surg 1973;60:646–9.
135. Malinchoc M, Kamath PS, Gordon FD, et al. A model to predict poor survival in patients undergoing transjugular intrahepatic portosystemic shunts. Hepatology 2000;31:864–71.
136. Oellerich M, Burdelski M, Lautz HU, et al. Predictors of one-year pretransplant survival in patients with cirrhosis. Hepatology 1991;14:1029–34.
137. Propst A, Propst T, Zangerl G, et al. Prognosis and life expectancy in chronic liver disease. Dig Dis Sci 1995;40:1805–15.
138. Infante-Rivard C, Esnaola S, Villeneuve JP. Clinical and statistical validity of conventional prognostic factors in predicting short-term survival among cirrhotics. Hepatology 1987;7:660–4.
139. Lucey MR, Brown KA, Everson GT, et al. Minimal criteria for placement of adults on the liver transplant waiting list: a report of a national conference organized by the American Society of Transplant Physicians and the American Association for the Study of Liver Diseases. Liver Transpl Surg 1997;3:628–37.
140. Kamath PS, Wiesner RH, Malinchoc M, et al. A model to predict survival in patients with end-stage liver disease. Hepatology 2001;33:464–70.

141. Wiesner R, Edwards E, Freeman R, et al. Model for end-stage liver disease (MELD) and allocation of donor livers. Gastroenterology 2003;124:91–6.
142. Freeman RB, Wiesner RH, Edwards E, et al. Results of the first year of the new liver allocation plan. Liver Transpl 2004;10:7–15.
143. Murray KF, Carithers RL Jr, AASLD. AASLD practice guidelines: evaluation of the patient for liver transplantation. Hepatology 2005;41:1407–32.
144. Fattovich G, Giustina G, Degos F, et al. Morbidity and mortality in compensated cirrhosis type C: a retrospective follow-up study of 384 patients. Gastroenterology 1997;112:463–72.
145. D'Amico G, Garcia-Tsao G, Pagliaro L. Natural history and prognostic indicators of survival in cirrhosis: a systematic review of 118 studies. J Hepatol 2006;44: 217–31.
146. Dienstag JL, Ghany MG, Morgan TR, et al. A prospective study of the rate of progression in compensated, histologically advanced chronic hepatitis C. Hepatology 2011;54:396–405.

When to Consider Liver Transplant During the Management of Chronic Liver Disease

Rena K. Fox, MD, FACP

KEYWORDS

- Liver transplantation • Chronic liver disease • Cirrhosis • Referral • Timing
- Clinical practice • Primary care • Evaluation

KEY POINTS

- The increasing prevalence of chronic liver disease and increasing prevalence of cirrhosis and hepatocellular carcinoma will bring an increasing demand for liver transplantation.
- Improved education and a simple guide for primary physicians are necessary for a timely referral of patients for liver transplant evaluation.
- Long-term management of patients with cirrhosis should include a regular repeated calculation of the Model for End-Stage Liver Disease (MELD) score to continually assess the appropriate time for transplant referral.
- Patients with a MELD score of 15 or greater should be referred for transplant, and Ideally at a score of 10 or greater to allow adequate time for evaluation.
- Any patient with cirrhosis should be referred for liver transplantation evaluation at the time of their first decompensating event, regardless of MELD.

INTRODUCTION

The rising prevalence of cirrhosis in the United States is alarming. Models predict that within 40 to 50 years, the peak incidence of end-stage liver disease due to hepatitis C virus (HCV) will be 38,000 and the peak prevalence of cirrhosis due to HCV in the US will be 1 million, and that by 2060, one-third of the HCV infected population will die of HCV if untreated. These estimates only refer to liver disease due to HCV, so including other causes of liver disease make these numbers even higher.[1,2] In the United States, liver cirrhosis is currently the 12th most common cause of death (9.5/100,000 individuals). Examining these statistics, it is predicted that over the next several decades there will

Disclosures: No relationships to disclose.
Division of General Internal Medicine, Department of Medicine, University of California, San Francisco School of Medicine, 1545 Divisadero Street, Suite 307, San Francisco, CA 94143-0320, USA
E-mail address: rfox@medicine.ucsf.edu

Med Clin N Am 98 (2014) 153–168
http://dx.doi.org/10.1016/j.mcna.2013.09.007
0025-7125/14/$ – see front matter © 2014 Elsevier Inc. All rights reserved.

be a rapid increase in the demand for liver transplantation (LT). At present, HCV infection is the leading indication for LT in the United States,[3] and as the HCV population is aging and the number of patients developing cirrhosis from HCV increases, the demand for LT as a result of HCV is expected to increase.[1] However, with the rising prevalence of the metabolic syndrome, it is staggering that approximately 30% to 40% of the United States population[4,5] is estimated to have nonalcoholic fatty liver disease (NAFLD). Although NAFLD has a much more benign course compared with HCV for most patients, approximately 30% with isolated steatosis will progress to nonalcoholic steatohepatitis (NASH). Of those with NASH, a small but significant proportion will progress to more serious liver disease. It is estimated that 20% of NASH patients will develop cirrhosis and approximately one-third of the cirrhotics will decompensate.[6,7] NAFLD has already grown to be the fourth most common reason for LT.[8] It is anticipated that NASH will potentially become the leading indication for transplantation as more effective treatments for HCV become available and the prevalence of cirrhosis from NAFLD increases.[8,9] Although local access to subspecialists has been shown to be associated with the likelihood of receiving a transplant,[10] with the astounding prevalence of the metabolic syndrome and diabetes,[11] many more of these patients will be managed in the primary care setting and may not have access to gastroenterology and hepatology specialists locally. One can thus expect primary care physicians to be increasingly making the diagnosis of chronic liver disease or cirrhosis, and the decision of when to refer their patients for LT evaluation.

KEEPING AN EYE ON TRANSPLANT TIMING DURING LONG-TERM MANAGEMENT OF CIRRHOSIS

Every chronic liver disease can eventually progress to cirrhosis, although some liver diseases are more likely than others to lead to cirrhosis. Because patients with chronic liver disease are almost always asymptomatic, physicians must actively watch for and recognize cirrhosis when it develops. The diagnosis of cirrhosis is not always straightforward[12]; and it is often misunderstood. Mistakenly, many physicians rely on serum aminotransferase levels, although both alanine aminotransferase and serum bilirubin have been shown to be nonpredictive of a diagnosis of cirrhosis.[12] Regularly reassessing all patients with chronic liver disease for any signs of cirrhosis is a major task for the primary care clinician, and education and understanding of the early signs and symptoms is lacking.[13] Patients and physicians may not be aware of development of cirrhosis during asymptomatic phases.

Cirrhosis itself is a progressive disease that results ultimately in death unless transplant is available (**Fig. 1**).[14–17] The median survival of patients with compensated cirrhosis is greater than 12 years and the median survival of those with decompensated cirrhosis is approximately 2 years.[17] The transition from a compensated to a decompensated phase occurs at a rate of approximately 5% to 7% per year and can be divided into stages. Stage 1 cirrhosis is characterized by an absence of esophageal varices and ascites. Stage 2 cirrhotics have developed esophagogastric varices without bleeding, but still have an absence of ascites. The presence of ascites signals stage 3 disease, which may or may not be associated with varices without bleeding. Stage 4 cirrhotics have developed gastrointestinal bleeding with or without the presence of ascites. Stages 1 and 2 are compensated stages, whereas stages 3 and 4 are decompensated stages. Ascites is the most common first presentation of decompensation. The mortality rate in stage 1 is 1% per year; however, patients progress from stage 1 at a cumulative rate of 11.4% per year, moving into either stage 2 or directly to stage 3. The mortality rate in stage 2 cirrhosis is 3.4% per year, progressing to either

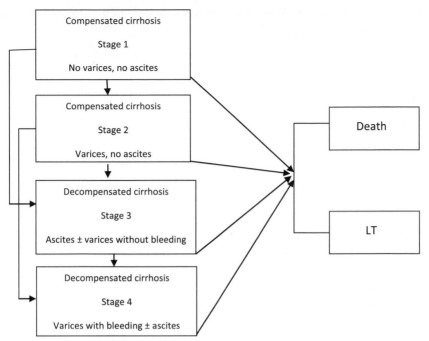

Fig. 1. Cirrhosis progression leads to either liver transplantation (LT) or death.

stage 3 or directly to stage 4. The stage 3 mortality rate is 20% per year, which actually far exceeds the rate of progression to stage 4. The stage 4 mortality rate is 57%, and nearly half of these deaths occur within 6 weeks of the initial episode of bleeding. Additionally, heptocellular carcinoma (HCC) develops at a rate of 3% per year, but it is not a unique stage of cirrhosis or defined as a decompensating event.[17] Understanding the usual course of disease progression in a cirrhotic patient is a necessity for primary care physicians.

Long-term management of cirrhotic patients includes regularly assessing the stage of cirrhosis and considering appropriate timing for a transplant referral, or referral to specialist for consultation and comanagement before the time of transplant referral.[18] Although integration of a specialist for every patient with cirrhosis would be ideal, the supply and distribution of specialists and subspecialists will never be adequate to cover all patients with cirrhosis. The primary management responsibility will ultimately rest with the primary care physician. However, the timing of transplant referral is often left out of the medical training on cirrhosis care, and even published guidelines on the management of cirrhosis do not always include transplant referral as part of their recommendations.[19]

Despite significant improvements in the medical management of cirrhosis and its complications, patients still suffer a reduced quality of life. Patients and physicians must prepare for the fact that cirrhosis will inevitably progress to liver failure and death, and that as survival times rapidly decrease for patients once they enter the decompensated phase, and that LT is the only definitive option in this setting.

GOALS AND SUCCESS OF LIVER TRANSPLANTATION

The goals of liver transplantation are to prolong quality of life and survival in patients with cirrhosis, end-stage liver disease, and HCC. Over the past 2 decades, liver transplantation has evolved from an experimental procedure to becoming the standard of care for many patients with end-stage liver disease. The remarkable increase in transplants over the past 2 decades has had a beneficial effect on the mortality from chronic liver disease in the United States.[20] As of June 2012 there were 17,000 patients on the LT waiting list, with more than 5000 transplantations performed. As transplantation has evolved, there are increasingly higher rates of survival and longer survival. In the United States, 1-, 3-, and 5-year survival rates are 87%, 80%, and 73% respectively. In addition, the quality of life after LT has improved greatly over the years.[21]

DISPARITIES IN THE USE OF LIVER TRANSPLANTATION

Disparities exist in many facets of medical care, but are even more pronounced in the area of LT. Multiple groups of patients have lower access to LT and lower rates of receiving a transplant. The Model for End-Stage Liver Disease (MELD) score for listing patients was adopted in 2002. Before this, compared to white patients, black patients were underrepresented on the waiting list, had more advanced disease at listing, and were more likely to die while awaiting LT. These differences are not seen in the MELD era.[22] However, certain minority populations, including Hispanic and Asian transplant candidates, are listed for transplant at more advanced stages of disease and have higher MELD scores at the time of listing.[23] Patients with Medicare and Medicaid, in comparison with patients with private insurance, have higher MELD scores at the time of listing and lower survival rates after transplantation.[24] Women have lower rates of LT than men. Female gender has been associated with an approximate 15% increased risk of death on the waiting list and a 12% decrease in the probability of receiving LT.[25,26] In comparison with patients with a diagnosis of viral hepatitis, patients with alcoholic cirrhosis are approximately half as likely to be listed for liver transplantation.[27]

INDICATIONS FOR LIVER TRANSPLANTATION

Transplantation should be considered for any patient when the life expectancy is shorter without a transplant than with a transplant, or when a transplant will likely improve the quality of life. By far the most common indication for transplant is end-stage liver disease as a result of chronic liver diseases, and currently HCV is the leading indication. Outside of end-stage liver disease, indications include HCC as well as other primary hepatobiliary malignancies. In addition, acute liver failure of any cause is an indication for transplantation if the patient is neurologically intact, psychosocially stable, and otherwise medically well enough for surgery. Another group of patients are those without end-stage liver disease but with recurrent life-threatening complications relating to liver disease (eg, recurrent cholangitis). This review focuses on when to consider LT during the management of chronic liver disease, and outcomes of chronic liver disease in adults (**Box 1**).

ABSOLUTE CONTRAINDICATIONS TO LIVER TRANSPLANTATION
Cardiac and Pulmonary Diseases

Most centers require a complete cardiopulmonary evaluation of all patients before listing for liver transplantation. Dobutamine stress echocardiography is an effective screening test for occult coronary disease in this setting.[28,29] Patients with positive tests should undergo cardiac catheterization to define the extent and to potentially treat existing coronary disease.

Box 1
Chronic liver diseases indicated for transplant

Chronic Noncholestatic Liver Disorders

Chronic hepatitis C

Chronic hepatitis B

Autoimmune hepatitis

Alcoholic liver disease

Nonalcoholic fatty liver disease

Cholestatic Liver Disorders

Primary biliary cirrhosis

Primary sclerosing cholangitis

Biliary atresia

Alagille syndrome

Metabolic Liver Disease

α1-Antitrypsin deficiency

Wilson disease

Hereditary hemochromatosis

Glycogen storage disease types I and IV

Neonatal hemochromatosis

Hemophilia A and B

Vascular Diseases of the Liver

Budd-Chiari syndrome

Veno-occlusive disease

Primary Malignancies of the Liver

Hepatocellular carcinoma

Cholangiocarcinoma

Hepatoblastoma

Hemangioendothelioma

Acute Liver Failure

Hepatitis A

Autoimmune hepatitis

Hepatitis B

Hepatitis C

Acute fatty liver of pregnancy

Reyes syndrome

Drugs (acetaminophen)

Miscellaneous Conditions

Polycystic liver disease

Severe graft-versus-host disease

Amyloidosis

Sarcoidosis

Hepatic trauma

Nodular regenerative hyperplasia

Sepsis or Active Infection

Although infection such as cholangitis or bacterial peritonitis is frequently related to progressive liver disease, active infection would threaten a successful transplant, especially with the onset of immunosuppression after transplant.

Extrahepatic Malignancy

Extrahepatic malignancies would be an absolute contraindication. However, patients with a history of a malignancy usually will be still be considered for LT if the malignancy occurred 2 to 5 years before transplant evaluation, depending on the specific malignancy.[30]

AIDS-Defining Illness or Poorly Controlled Human Immunodeficiency Virus

Well-controlled human immunodeficiency virus (HIV) is not a contraindication, but AIDS-defining illnesses or unresponsive or uncontrolled HIV would have a high risk of poor outcome after transplant.

Inadequate Social Support

Issues that would prevent the logistic life accommodations necessary to fulfill the commitment of maintaining posttransplant care, or patients with psychosocial barriers to full compliance or who lack adequate social support, would be poor candidates for transplantation. Severe psychiatric disorders that might impede medical compliance would place the patient at risk for proper care after transplant.

Active Substance Use

Active substance abuse, including the use of alcohol, is generally considered to be a contraindication to transplantation. Patients who are actively using alcohol or drugs have higher rates of medical noncompliance and failure to adhere to recommendations after transplantation. Patients with a history of alcohol abuse must generally meet 6 months of absolute abstinence, often in addition to successful completion of an alcohol rehabilitation program. The 6-month rule of abstinence is not uniform but is generally followed in United States and European transplant programs.[31]

RELATIVE CONTRAINDICATIONS TO LIVER TRANSPLANTATION

The list of relative contraindications varies between centers, and the considerations for these issues are currently evolving.

Advanced Age

Advanced age is not a contraindication for liver transplantation, but as the age of transplant recipients rises there is concern for increases in complications, particularly from cardiopulmonary diseases. Most centers have an age cutoff between 65 and 70 years, although many centers do not use a fixed limit and would consider an older patient if the individual would otherwise have good life expectancy.[32,33]

Obesity

Obesity poses multiple problems for patients in terms of technical problems of surgery and higher incidence of postsurgical complications. Most transplant centers have a body mass index (BMI) cutoff of 40 kg/m^2, although other centers may also consider a BMI of greater than 35 kg/m^2 to be prohibitive.[34]

HIV Infection

HIV was previously an absolute contraindication to transplantation. However, HIV is not now a contraindication in and of itself. HIV disease must be well controlled, however, to consider LT. Most centers do not yet perform transplantation for patients with HIV infection, but a few centers do. HIV must be well controlled (negative viral load and CD4 counts >250).[35,36]

Malnutrition

Low body weight, particularly BMI less than 19 to 20 kg/m^2 at the time of transplantation, is a poor prognostic factor for transplant outcome.

History of Poor Medical Adherence

Patients with poor medical compliance may not be able to perform the necessary medication regimen and follow-up regimen in the posttransplant period, and thus may suffer from poor outcomes after transplantation.

IMPORTANCE OF TIMING OF INITIAL REFERRAL

The appropriate timing of the initial referral for transplant evaluation is critical for optimal individual patient care as well as for a functioning transplant system as a whole. Referral is the first step in an extensive evaluation process and waiting-list period. Therefore, referral must take place when a patient is well enough to undergo evaluation and listing, but sick enough to have developed the signs of progression to a terminal state.

Originally, the organ allocation policy was determined on first-come first-served basis and was highly problematic. Prioritization was based on cumulative wait-list time, resulting in some patients being registered earlier than needed but accumulating priority with long waiting times. Patients most in need based on severity would be listed with a lower priority than less ill patients who were already waiting on the list for longer times. The first attempt to change this policy was made by the United Network for Organ Sharing (UNOS), stratifying patients based on disease severity according to the intensity of the care the patient was receiving, such as intensive care unit in comparison with ambulatory care. However, these were vague boundaries and that varied according to regional differences in medical practices.

In the current era, need-based listing has required the development of objective criteria to guide the appropriate time for referral. These criteria can be non–disease-specific recommendations, focusing on severity of cirrhosis, regardless of the etiology of the liver disease, or disease-specific recommendations related to the underlying condition.

Timing Based on Severity of End-Stage Liver Disease

Determining the appropriate timing to refer a patient for transplant can be based on the severity of liver disease. Severity can be determined by calculation of the MELD score, determination of the Child-Turcotte-Pugh (CTP) score, or by identification of cirrhosis complications. Published guidelines from the American Association for the Study of Liver Diseases (AASLD) refer to all 3 as ways to determine the time for initial referral.[36]

Model for End-Stage Liver Disease Score

The MELD score was originally developed to predict short-term (3 months) prognosis in patients undergoing transjugular intrahepatic portosystemic shunts (TIPS).[37,38] It is a mathematical score determined using 3 clinical laboratory measurements: serum creatinine, International Normalized Ratio (INR), and total bilirubin. These factors were observed to have a statistical impact on patient mortality. Under the MELD model, patients are scored from 6 to 40, on a continuous scale. The MELD score equates to 3-month survival rates (**Table 1**). Over time, MELD has been validated as predictive of prognosis of patients with chronic liver disease at various time points, and in patients with different severities and causes of liver disease, and from different geographic origins.[38]

MELD has been instituted as a prioritization tool for the LT waiting list since 2002, with the highest MELD scores being treated with the highest priority.[39] This policy was based on the finding that survival while on the waiting list correlated with the MELD score at the time of placement on the waiting list.[40,41]

The implementation of MELD-based policy on the transplant system has shown an impressive impact. Findings include a decrease in new registrations on the waiting list as a result of reduced importance in overall waiting time, a decrease in wait-list mortality, a decrease in rate of removal from the waiting list because of progression of disease severity, an increase in organ availability, a decrease in the median waiting time to orthotopic LT, an overall increase in the rate of transplants performed, an increase in patient survival rate after transplantation, and an increase in graft survival rate after transplantation.[40]

The benefits of MELD as a score are also in its simplicity and objectivity. Each variable is a readily available laboratory value, and there is no subjectivity in assessment of clinical disease. The variables are not weighted equally; rather, each variable is weighted according to its effect on prognosis. The score is also independent of the type of liver disease.

The MELD score also has limitations and weaknesses. It is well recognized that there are complications of cirrhosis that can affect quality of life and survival but may not be reflected in the calculated MELD score, such as hyponatremia,[42] malnutrition, and complications of portal hypertension. The impact of these issues is being

Table 1
Model for End-Stage Liver Disease (MELD)

MELD Equation[a]:
MELD = 3.78[Ln serum bilirubin (mg/dL)] + 11.2[Ln INR] + 9.57[Ln serum creatinine (mg/dL)] + 6.43
where INR is International Normalized Ratio
If the patient has been dialyzed twice within the last 7 days, the value for serum creatinine used should be 4.0
Any value less than 1 is given a value of 1

Score	3-Month Mortality (%)[b]
$\geq$40	71.3
30–39	52.6
20–29	19.6
10–19	6.0
<9	1.9

[a] *Data from* Available at: http://optn.transplant.hrsa.gov/resources/MeldPeldCalculator.asp?index=98. Accessed June 30, 2013.
[b] Wiesner R, Edwards E, Freeman R, et al. Model for end-stage liver disease (MELD) and allocation of donor livers. Gastroenterology 2003;124(1):91–6. PMID: 12512033.

studied with potential modifications to the MELD score to account for their existence. Gender has been identified as a factor that may be unequally addressed by MELD. It is notable that women have a decreased survival compared with men while waiting for a transplant. Because creatinine levels are related to muscle mass, women can have a lower creatinine level than men with the same glomerular filtration rate (GFR). Because the MELD score uses creatinine but not GFR, women and men could have similar MELD scores but women could be substantially sicker.[26] Moreover, although the MELD score relies only on laboratory values, there is variability between laboratories in the measurement of creatinine, INR, and bilirubin (see **Table 1**).

It is also recognized that there are comorbid conditions associated with cirrhosis that could change survival but would not be reflected in the calculated MELD score. These comorbidities include the presence of HCC, refractory upper variceal bleeding, refractory ascites and/or pleural effusions when TIPS is contraindicated, biliary strictures, recurrent biliary sepsis, severe polycystic liver disease, hepatopulmonary syndrome, and portopulmonary hypertension. To account for these conditions, adjustments to the calculated MELD score are performed by adding exception points depending on the condition.[43] Exception points allow MELD scores to increase to values that will allow these patients to undergo transplantation within a predictable time frame.

After implementation of the MELD score, it was shown that patients with MELD score of greater than 15 had greater mortality from their liver disease than from the mortality of undergoing liver transplantation, whereas patients with scores less than 15 showed a greater mortality risk from the transplant procedure and posttransplant state than from their liver disease left without a transplant.[44-46] Because of this finding, it is often recommended that physicians refer patients when their MELD reaches 15 or higher.[47,48] However, the AASLD recommendation that patients with a MELD score lower than 15, specifically a MELD of 10 or higher, be referred to allow for the usual time needed for the transplant evaluation (**Box 2**).[36] It is also recommended that referral be expedited for patients with complications that imminently threaten survival (**Box 3**).

Child-Turcotte-Pugh Score

The CTP classification was designed to stratify the risk of portacaval shunt surgery in patients with cirrhosis and variceal bleeding.[49] Over time, the CTP system also became widely used to classify the severity of chronic liver disease. The CTP score is composed of 3 laboratory variables, serum albumin, serum bilirubin, and serum prothrombin time, and 2 clinical variables, ascites and encephalopathy. The CTP score was never formally validated as a prognostic tool, yet survival data have shown that for patients with CTP scores of 10 or more (class C) who are waiting for LT, 1 year survival was 45%, for CTP scores of 7–9 (class B), 1 year survival was 84%, and for CTP scores of 5–6 (class A), 1 year survival was 81%.[50]

Box 2
Criteria for transplantation referral for chronic liver disease

CTP ≥7

MELD ≥10

First complication of cirrhosis: ascites, variceal bleeding, hepatic encephalopathy

According to the AASLD and American Society of Transplant Physicians.

Box 3
Conditions warranting expedited transplantation referral

Fulminant hepatic failure (critical care management)

Hepatopulmonary syndrome

Hepatorenal syndrome type I

The Organ Procurement and Transplantation Network (OPTN) initially used the CTP score along with waiting time to define the listing priority based on UNOS criteria before the MELD system was implemented. Multiple studies have since demonstrated the superiority of MELD over CTP in predicting short-term mortality on the waiting list.[51–53] Nonetheless, the benefits of CTP have kept its position as part of the assessment of patients with cirrhosis. The CTP score is much more widely known by nonspecialists and has been in practice much longer than MELD. The CTP score is simple to use. In addition, as a categorical scale rather than a continuous scale, there are only a few classes for patients to fit into; this limits its performance as a tool to prioritize patients on the waiting list. Finally, the CTP score does not consider renal function, which is an independent predictor of survival in patients with end-stage liver disease.[54]

Assessment of CTP score is still included in recommendations for transplant evaluation,[55] and the AASLD recommends if CTP is used, that an initial transplant referral be considered when a patient's CTP score is greater than or equal to 7 (see **Box 2**).[36]

Evidence of Decompensated Cirrhosis

In patients with cirrhosis, the transition from compensated to decompensated cirrhosis represents a major turning point in their prognosis. Complications include ascites, hepatic encephalopathy, hepatorenal syndrome, variceal bleeding, hepatopulmonary syndrome, or portopulmonary hypertension. Most commonly, ascites is the first complication. The 5-year survival rate when any of these complications develop is 20% to 50% of that in patients who are compensated.[56,57] The development of any of these complications indicates a movement out of stage 1 or stage 2 of cirrhosis, meaning that patients enter the phase of decompensation.

The AASLD guidelines include a recommendation to refer at the time of the first development of any decompensation event[36]; for example, referring a patient with previously compensated cirrhosis who then develops their first episode of ascites. Having a patient with uncomplicated ascites already referred for transplant allows the center to have prospective follow-up, and if refractory ascites, hyponatremia, spontaneous bacterial peritonitis, or hepatorenal syndrome develop, the patient can be closely managed on the waiting list. Acute liver failure, hepatopulmonary syndrome, and hepatorenal syndrome warrant expedited referral because of the high mortality rates once these conditions develop (see **Box 3**).

TIMING BASED ON THE SPECIFIC UNDERLYING LIVER DISEASE
Hepatocellular Carcinoma

Primary care physicians are the major group that can carry out the recommendations for HCC screening in appropriate patients: all patients with cirrhosis and with hepatitis B virus infection, and those in additional high-risk categories.[58,59] In addition, this means that primary care physicians are most likely to make the initial diagnosis of

HCC in asymptomatic patients who are undergoing screening. Understanding that liver transplantation is a treatment option for HCC is critical for primary care physicians.

Liver transplantation is indicated in patients with HCC that fits within the Milan criteria (a single nodule between 2 and 5 cm, or no more than 3 lesions, the largest of which is less than 3 cm, with no evidence of macrovascular invasion or metastasis). Some centers, with the permission of UNOS, apply expanded size criteria developed by the University of California, San Francisco to determine whether larger tumors can be successfully transplanted. In addition, tumors initially outside of size limitations may be reduced in size by chemoembolization or radiofrequency ablation to fit within these criteria. It is most important that primary care physicians or nontransplant gastroenterologists discuss each case, even for small tumors, with their referral center because centers may vary in their approach and in the criteria they use.

In HCC patients with compensated cirrhosis and low calculated MELD score, MELD exception points are granted to perform transplantation before tumors have had time to progress outside of transplantable criteria.

Cholangiocarcinoma

Patients with cholangiocarcinoma (CCA) were previously considered to have poor survival, and CCA was considered a transplant contraindication. Intrahepatic CCA is still a contraindication to LT,[60] but protocols combining chemoradiation and LT for hilar CCA have shown good survival rates.

Primary Biliary Cirrhosis and Primary Sclerosing Cholangitis

The Mayo Clinic developed models specific for primary biliary cirrhosis (PBC) and primary sclerosing cholangitis (PSC) to determine adequate time for referral. Recommendations have been that a Mayo risk score predicting greater than 10% mortality at 1 year without transplantation would be an indication for referral.[61] In addition, quality-of-life issues such as intractable pruritus, recurrent cholangitis, xanthomatous neuropathy, and severe metabolic bone disease may also be considered potential indications for transplantation in these specific settings.

ROLES FOR THE REFERRING PHYSICIAN IN OPTIMIZING PATIENTS FOR TRANSPLANT REFERRAL

Considering when a patient is appropriate for LT should include consideration of how to optimize the patient's likelihood of being a transplant candidate. Modifiable factors that may influence the patient's likelihood of receiving a transplant can be identified and addressed either before or after transplant referral (**Box 4**). Efforts toward sustained alcohol abstinence can be emphasized by referring physicians, to help prepare the patient in this regard to thus demonstrate their sobriety. Smoking is also a modifiable factor that can be addressed to ready a patient for optimal transplant eligibility. The use of prescription opiates, if poorly controlled and poorly adherent, can be another area to target before a patient reaches the need for a transplant referral. Obesity, an ever more prevalent disease, should be especially targeted for patients as their cirrhosis advances, not only because steatosis will hasten any liver disease but also because of BMI limits for transplant. Cardiovascular health can and should be optimized as much as possible for general fitness, but also with an eye toward candidacy for transplant. Finally, social support should be bolstered and confirmed.

Box 4
Factors potentially modifiable by referring physician to optimize patient's candidacy for transplant

Obesity

Alcohol use

Illicit drug use

Cigarette smoking

Social support

Medical adherence

Osteoporosis

Coronary artery disease

Pulmonary disease

Portopulmonary hypertension

Human immunodeficiency virus infection

Hepatitis C virus infection

Hepatitis B virus infection

Depression and anxiety

Chronic opioid use

Diabetes mellitus

Hyperlipidemia

SUMMARY

The decision to perform liver transplantation for a particular patient is never the decision of one single individual, although a single individual could preclude transplant as an option if the opportunity for referral is missed. Every physician treating patients with cirrhosis, including primary care physicians and primary gastroenterologists, should watch for the essential turning points at which a patient may become eligible for a transplant referral. Timing of referral could be assessed according to either the type of liver disease or non–disease-specific measures of disease severity. Although the MELD score is an easily accessible and convenient tool it is not as well known as CTP classification, and many cirrhotic patients under long-term management may not be being allocated a MELD score regularly calculated by their primary physicians. Because a slow progression in MELD score may occur without a change in symptoms, reaching the MELD score acceptable for transplant referral may go unrecognized.

As generalists face the rising prevalence of NAFLD and the rising prevalence of cirrhosis and HCC from HCV, there will be an increasing need for education in the management of liver disease. It will be necessary for specialists and health care systems to better inform primary care physicians about the recommendations on criteria for transplant referral and the critical windows of opportunity within which they can act. Although there is a recognized knowledge gap[13] that needs to be addressed, once a patient is in medical care, inadequate physician knowledge should never be the cause for late timing or missing the opportunity for referral.

REFERENCES

1. Rein DB, Wittenborn JS, Weinbaum CM, et al. Forecasting the morbidity and mortality associated with prevalent cases of pre-cirrhotic chronic hepatitis C in the United States. Dig Liver Dis 2011;43(1):66–72.
2. David GL, Alter MJ, El-Serag H, et al. Aging of hepatitis C virus (HCV)-infected persons in the United States: a multiple cohort model of HCV prevalence and disease progression. Gastroenterology 2010;138(2):513–21.
3. Curry MP. Hepatitis B and hepatitis C viruses in liver transplantation. Transplantation 2004;78(7):955–63.
4. Williams CD, Stengel J, Asike MI, et al. Prevalence of nonalcoholic fatty liver disease and nonalcoholic steatohepatitis among a largely middle-aged population utilizing ultrasound and liver biopsy: a prospective study. Gastroenterology 2011;140:124–31.
5. Browning JD, Szczepaniak LS, Dobbins R, et al. Prevalence of hepatic steatosis in an urban population in the United States: impact of ethnicity. Hepatology 2004;40:1387–95.
6. Levene AP, Goldin RD. The epidemiology, pathogenesis and histopathology of fatty liver disease. Histopathology 2012;61:141–52.
7. Chalasani N, Younossi Z, Lavine JE, et al. The diagnosis and management of non-alcoholic fatty liver disease: practice Guideline by the American Association for the Study of Liver Diseases, American College of Gastroenterology, and the American Gastroenterological Association. Hepatology 2012;55(6): 2005–23.
8. Watt KD, Charlton MR. Metabolic syndrome and liver transplantation; a review and guide to management. J Hepatol 2010;53:199–206.
9. Afzali A, Berry K, Ioannou GN. Excellent posttransplant survival for patients with nonalcoholic steatohepatitis in the United States. Liver Transpl 2012;18(1): 29–37.
10. Barritt AS IV, Telloni SA, Potter CW, et al. Local access to subspecialty care influences the chance of receiving a liver transplant. Liver Transpl 2013;19: 377–82.
11. US Center for Disease Control and Prevention. Vital statistics of the United States. Hyattsville (MD): National Center for Health Statistics; 1988. Mortality, 1988–2006.
12. Udell JA, Wang CS, Tinmouth J, et al. Does this patient with liver disease have cirrhosis? JAMA 2012;307(8):832–42.
13. Mitchell AE, Colvin HM, Palmer Beasley R. Institute of Medicine recommendations for the prevention and control of hepatitis B and C. Hepatology 2010; 51(3):729–33.
14. D'Amico G, Morabito A, Pagliaro L, et al. Survival and prognostic indicators in compensated and decompensated cirrhosis. Dig Dis Sci 1986;31:468–75.
15. Schepis F, Cammà C, Niceforo D, et al. Which patients with cirrhosis should undergo endoscopic screening for esophageal varices detection? Hepatology 2001;33(2):333–8.
16. Garcia-Tsao G, Friedman S, Iredale J, et al. Now there are many (stages) where before there was one: in search of a pathophysiological classification of cirrhosis. Hepatology 2010;51(4):1445–9.
17. D'Amico G, Garcia-Tsao G, Pagliaro L. Natural history and prognostic indicators of survival in cirrhosis: a systematic review of 118 studies. J Hepatol 2006;44: 217–31.

18. Grattagliano I, Ubaldi E, Bonfrate L, et al. Management of liver cirrhosis between primary care and specialists. World J Gastroenterol 2011;17(18):2273–82.

19. Garcia-Tsao G, Lim JK, Members of Veterans Affairs Hepatitis C Resource Center Program. Management and treatment of patients with cirrhosis and portal hypertension: recommendations from the Department of Veterans Affairs Hepatitis C Resource Center Program and the National Hepatitis C Program. Am J Gastroenterol 2009;104:1802–29.

20. Evans RW. Liver transplants and the decline in deaths from liver disease. Am J Public Health 1997;87:868–9.

21. Availalble at: http://optn.transplant.hrsa.gov/latestData/rptStrat.asp. Accessed October 15, 2013.

22. Moylan CA, Brady CW, Johnson JL, et al. Disparities in liver transplantation before and after introduction of the MELD score. JAMA 2008;300(20):2371–8.

23. Mathur AK, Schaubel DE, Gong Q, et al. Racial and ethnic disparities in access to liver transplantation. Liver Transpl 2010;16(9):1033–40.

24. Bryce CL, Angus DC, Arnold RM, et al. Sociodemographic differences in early access to liver transplantation services. Am J Transplant 2009;9(9):2092–101.

25. Lai JC, Terrault NA, Vittinghoff E, et al. Height contributes to the gender difference in wait-list mortality under the MELD-based liver allocation system. Am J Transplant 2010;10(12):2658–64.

26. Myers RP, Shaheen AA, Aspinall AI, et al. Gender, renal function, and outcomes on the liver transplant waiting list: assessment of revised MELD including estimated glomerular filtration rate. J Hepatol 2011;54(3):462–70.

27. Julapalli VR, Kramer JR, El-Serag HB. Evaluation for liver transplantation: adherence to AASLD referral guidelines in a large Veterans Affairs center. Liver Transpl 2005;11:1370–8.

28. Donovan CL, Marcovitz PA, Punch JD, et al. Two-dimensional and dobutamine stress echocardiography in the preoperative assessment of patients with end-stage liver disease prior to orthotopic liver transplantation. Transplantation 1996;61:1180–8.

29. Williams K, Lewis JF, Davis G, et al. Dobutamine stress echocardiography in patients undergoing liver transplantation evaluation. Transplantation 2000;69:2354–6.

30. Alqahtani S. Update in liver transplantation. Curr Opin Gastroenterol 2012;28:230–8.

31. Lim JK, Keeffe EB. Liver transplantation for alcoholic liver disease: current concepts and length of sobriety. Liver Transpl 2004;10(10 Suppl 2):S31–8.

32. Keswani RN, Ahmed A, Keeffe EB. Older age and liver transplantation: a review. Liver Transpl 2004;10(8):957–67.

33. Lipshutz GS, Busuttil RW. Liver transplantation in those of advancing age: the case for transplantation. Liver Transpl 2007;13(10):1355–7.

34. Nair S, Verma S, Thuluvath PJ. Obesity and its effect on survival in patients undergoing orthotopic liver transplantation in the United States. Hepatology 2002;35(1):105–9.

35. Ahmed A, Keeffe EB. Current indications and contraindications for liver transplantation. Clin Liver Dis 2007;11:227–47.

36. Murray KF, Carithers RL. AASLD practice guidelines: evaluation of the patient for liver transplantation. Hepatology 2005;41(6):1407–32.

37. Malinchoc M, Kamath PS, Gordon FD, et al. A model to predict poor survival in patients undergoing transjugular intrahepatic portosystemic shunts. Hepatology 2000;31:864–71.

38. Kanath P. A model to predict survival in patients with end stage liver disease. Hepatology 2001;33:464–70.
39. Wiesner R, The United Network for Organ Sharing Liver Disease Severity Score Committee. Model for end-stage liver disease (MELD) and allocation of donor livers. Gastroenterology 2003;124:91.
40. Bernardi M. The MELD score in patients awaiting liver transplant: strengths and weaknesses. J Hepatol 2011;54:1297–306.
41. Freeman RB, Wiesner RH, Edwards E, et al. Results of the first year of the new liver allocation plan. Liver Transpl 2004;10:7–15.
42. Kim WR, Biggins SW. Hyponatremia and mortality among patients on the liver-transplant waiting list. N Engl J Med 2008;359:1018–26.
43. Freeman RB Jr, Gish RG, Harper A, et al. Model for end-stage liver disease (MELD) exception guidelines: results and recommendations from the MELD Exception Study Group and Conference (MESSAGE) for the approval of patients who need liver transplantation with diseases not considered by the standard MELD formula. Liver Transpl 2006;12(12 Suppl 3):S128–36.
44. Merion RM, Schaubel DE, Dykstra DM, et al. The survival benefit of liver transplantation. Am J Transplant 2005;5:307–13.
45. Martin AP, Bartels M, Hauss J, et al. Overview of the MELD score and the UNOS adult liver allocation system. Transplant Proc 2007;39(10):3169–74.
46. Hanto DW, Fishbein TM, Pinson CW, et al. Liver and intestine transplantation: summary analysis 1994-2003. Am J Transplant 2005;5:916–33.
47. Siciliano M. Liver transplantation in adults: choosing the appropriate timing. World J Gastrointest Pharmacol Ther 2012;3(4):49–61.
48. Starr SP, Raines D. Cirrhosis: diagnosis, management, and prevention. Am Fam Physician 2011;84(12):1353–9.
49. Pugh RN, Murray-Lyon IM, Dawson JL, et al. Transection of the oesophagus for bleeding varices. Br J Surg 1973;60:646–9.
50. Boin IF, Leonardi MI, Pinto RS, et al. Liver transplant recipients mortality on the waiting list: long-term comparison to child-pugh classification and MELD. Transplant Proc 2004;36(4):920–2.
51. Durand F, Valla D. Assessment of the prognosis of cirrhosis: child-Pugh versus MELD. J Hepatol 2005;42:S100–7.
52. Asrani SK, Kim WR. Model for end stage liver disease: end of the first decade. Clin Liver Dis 2011;15(4):685–98.
53. Cuomo O, Perrella A, Arenga G. Model for end-stage liver disease (MELD) score system to evaluate patients with viral hepatitis on the waiting list: better than the child-turcotte-pugh (CTP) system? Transplantation Proc 2008;40:1906–9.
54. Cooper GS, Bellamy P, Dawson NV, et al. A prognostic model for patients with end stage liver disease. Gastroenterology 1997;113:1278–88.
55. Lucey MR, Brown KA, Everson GT, et al. Minimal criteria for placement of adults on the liver transplant waiting list: a report of a national conference organized by the American Society of Transplant Physicians and the American Association for the Study of Liver Diseases. Liver Transpl Surg 1997;3(6):628–37.
56. Ginés P, Quintero E, Arroyo V, et al. Compensated cirrhosis: natural history and prognostic factors. Hepatology 1987;7:122–8.
57. Arsani SK, Kamath PS. Natural history of cirrhosis. Curr Gastroenterol Rep 2013; 15(2):308.
58. Lok AS, McMahon BJ. Chronic hepatitis B. Hepatology 2007;45:507–39.
59. Bruix J, Sherman M, American Association for the Study of Liver Diseases. Management of hepatocellular carcinoma: an update. Hepatology 2011;53(3):1020–2.

60. Ali JM, Bonomo L, Brais R, et al. Outcomes and diagnostic challenges posed by incidental cholangiocarcinoma after liver transplantation. Transplantation 2011; 91(12):1392–7.

61. Shetty K, Rybicki L, Carey WD. The Child-Pugh classification as a prognostic indicator for survival in primary sclerosing cholangitis. Hepatology 1997;25(5): 1049–53.

Index

Note: Page numbers of article titles are in **boldface** type.

A

Abdominal pain, in hepatocellular carcinoma, 106
Abscess, of liver, 108–109
N-Acetyl-cysteine, for NAFLD, 65
Adefovir, for hepatitis B, 47–48
Adenomas, hepatic, 108
ADVANCE study, for hepatitis C, 22–24
Age factors, in liver transplantation, 158
Alanine aminotransferase (ALT), 2–5
Albumin
    for ascites, 124
    for hepatorenal syndrome, 131
    for spontaneous bacterial peritonitis, 127–128
    measurement of, in ascites, 120
    synthesis of, 12–13
Alcoholic liver disease, aminotransferases in, 4, 6
Alisporovir, for hepatitis C, 33–34
Alkaline phosphatase, 5–8, 13
Alpha$_1$-antitrypsin deficiency, aminotransferases in, 6
Alpha-fetoprotein, in hepatocellular carcinoma, 104
Amebic abscess, 109
Amiloride, for ascites, 123
Aminotransferases, 2–5, 13
Ammonia, accumulation of, in hepatic encephalopathy, 137–138
Ammonium tetrathiomolybdate, for Wilson disease, 96–97
Angiotensin receptor blockers, for NAFLD, 65–66
Antibiotics
    for spontaneous bacterial peritonitis, 127–129
    for variceal bleeding, 136
    liver injury due to, cholestasis in, 7
Antimitochondrial antibodies, in cholestatic liver disease, 77
Antioxidants, for NAFLD, 64–65
Ascites, 120–132
    differential diagnosis of, 121
    dilutional hyponatremia in, 130
    evaluation of, 120–122
    gastrointestinal hemorrhage in, 129
    hepatorenal syndrome in, 130–131
    hydrothorax in, 132
    refractory, 123–124
    spontaneous bacterial peritonitis in, 125–129

Med Clin N Am 98 (2014) 169–180
http://dx.doi.org/10.1016/S0025-7125(13)00173-9
0025-7125/14/$ – see front matter © 2014 Elsevier Inc. All rights reserved.

medical.theclinics.com